The
Herbal
Healer

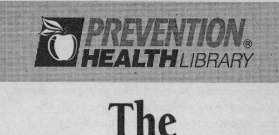

PREVENTION® HEALTH LIBRARY

The Herbal Healer

By the editors of

PREVENTION Health Books™

Rodale Press, Inc.
Emmaus, Pennsylvania

The information in this book is excerpted from *The Complete Book of Natural and Medicinal Cures* (Rodale Press, 1994).

Copyright © 1998 by Rodale Press, Inc.

Printed in the United States of America on acid-free ∞, recycled paper ♻

Cover and book designer: Diane Ness Shaw

ISBN 1-57954-089-9 paperback

2 4 6 8 10 9 7 5 3 1 paperback

OUR PURPOSE

"We inspire and enable people to improve their lives and the world around them."

Notice

This book is intended as a reference volume only, not as a medical manual. The information given here is designed to help you make informed decisions about your health. It is not intended as a substitute for any treatment that may have been prescribed by your doctor. If you suspect that you have a medical problem, we urge you to seek competent medical help.

Contents

For the best interactive guide to healthy active living,
visit our Web site at **http://www.healthyideas.com.**

Introduction

Healing Wisdom at Your Fingertips

Visit the shampoo aisle at your local grocery store. Stop by the corner drugstore. Look around the food mart at your neighborhood gas station. Turn on the TV. Everywhere you'll see mention of herbs. There are teas with ginseng. Shampoos with aloe. And herbal formulas to enhance your mood, soothe your nerves, sharpen your mind or provide a hundred other benefits.

Yes, herbs are popular these days—and with good reason: Research in this country and in Europe has shown again and again that herbs have proven power to heal. No longer is there a question of whether herbs are good for you; now, the question is which herbs work best for which conditions and in what doses.

That's where this book will help. Our editors at *Prevention Health Books* have spent months interviewing medical and herbal experts to find the most accurate information on 60 herbs that researchers believe may have potent healing potential. Read this book and you'll learn how each of these herbs works, the diseases or conditions each one may help relieve, the appropriate daily doses and the safest way to use each herb.

If you're in a hurry, you may want to turn to the handy Cure Finder at the front of the book to quickly find the right herbal remedy for more than 130 conditions, from allergies and anxiety, to ulcers and yeast infections.

Or if you'd like to learn what this "herb stuff" is all about, you can start with Part 1: A Guide to Nature's Drugstore, and learn the basics, including what terms like *essential oil*, *infusion* and *tincture* mean. In Part 2: Herbs That Heal, you'll discover A-to-Z listings and detailed explanations of all the herbs.

However you use the book, you're sure to find it entertaining and valuable. Enjoy the book and your exciting journey to greater health!

The Cure Finder

Finding Just the Right Remedies

PART 1

A Guide to Nature's Drugstore

Herbal Remedies

Nature's Practical Wisdom

Since the dawn of time, people have turned to plants for medicine. In fact, until this century, plant medicine, mingled with faith and luck, was just about the only medicine. Then came laboratories, scientists in white smocks and a host of powerful tablets and injections that grabbed the spotlight from leaves, roots, bark and berries. As dreaded diseases were conquered, many gentle and time-honored natural remedies were all but forgotten.

Now things seem to be coming full circle. Many people, seeking alternatives to the cost and side effects of synthetic medications, are turning back to herbs for all kinds of ailments.

But the revival of herbal medicine has brewed up a controversy hotter than a cup of chamomile tea. Are herbs an unexplored treasure trove of natural cures? Or are they a snake oil salesman's dream come true?

There is no easy answer to that question. Recent research shows that some herbs do, in fact, offer powerful medicinal benefits. Chances are there are many beneficial herbs as yet unresearched and not yet recognized by American medical authorities. But there are also a lot of extravagant claims made for herbs. And diagnosing and dosing yourself with herbs can be a dangerous game. In this section, we'll show you how to explore the potential benefits of herbs while steering clear of possible risks.

Plant Power

The simplest description of an herb is a "useful plant." Even in this day of high-tech drugs, plants continue to serve as potent and powerful healing agents. In the United States, about a quarter of all prescriptions contain active ingredients from plants, says Norman R. Farnsworth, Ph.D., director of the Program for Collaborative Research in the Pharmaceutical Sciences at the University of Illinois at Chicago.

For decades, plant-based medications such as digitalis (from the herb foxglove) for the heart and quinine (from the bark of the cinchona tree) for malaria have been saving lives. Joining them are newer drugs such as taxol, a potent cancer therapy derived from the Pacific yew, says John Beutler, Ph.D., a chemist with the National Cancer Institute. Dr. Beutler screens thousands of exotic plants each year for their cancer-fighting potential. "Plant medicines are not hokum," he says. "They offer real promise, but first scientists have to take a good, critical look at them."

Even the corner drugstore holds an herbal bouquet of familiar remedies. A wide variety of nonprescription products—from mentholated cough drops (derived from mint) to psyllium laxatives and witch hazel—contain real or synthesized plant substances. Technically, even a cup of coffee is a mild herbal stimulant.

For most of us, though, a mention of "herbs" conjures up plants with quaint names like feverfew and

3

An Herbal Glossary

Astringent: An agent that diminishes internal or external secretions or causes soft tissues to pucker.

Bitter: A substance that stimulates secretion of saliva and increases appetite.

Decoction: A water extract of herbs made by boiling or simmering; stronger than a tea.

Demulcent: A substance that soothes inflamed mucous membranes.

Digestive: Improving digestion.

Diuretic: Increasing flow of urine.

Elixir: An alcohol-based medication, usually sweetened.

Essential oil: A volatile (easily vaporized) and scented plant oil found in many herbal medications.

Expectorant: Easing the coughing up of mucus.

Infusion: A medication made by combining plants or plant extracts with boiling water; similar to a tea.

Mucilage: A sticky substance found in plants, used to soothe inflammation.

Poultice: A moist, hot compress applied externally to the body.

Simple: A medicinal herb without strong effects.

Tea: A dried substance, usually from a plant, steeped in hot water for drinking.

Tincture: A medication with its active agent dissolved in alcohol.

Tonic: An agent to maintain or restore health in one organ system or the whole body.

goldenseal, brewed up in teas and used in tinctures. Many of these plants have a long history of use, described in folklore of various cultures. It's possible that your own grandmothers used them.

In some cases, research has proved that the old-time herbalists were on the right track. "A fairly high percentage of useful plant-derived drugs were discovered as a result of scientific follow-up of well-known plants used in traditional medicine," says Dr. Farnsworth. Not all traditional herb uses stand up under strict scientific scrutiny, however. Some of them have proven to be ineffective or even toxic. And many simply haven't been thoroughly studied yet.

What Labels Don't Tell

If you have ever shopped for herbal products in a health food store, you may have noticed something odd: The labels almost never tell the potential medical benefits of the herb. And unlike standard medicines such as aspirin, most herbal remedies come without directions or precautions for use.

The reason? The Food and Drug Administration (FDA) prohibits manufacturers from making claims that any product will treat or prevent a disease until that product has been exhaustively tested.

Many herbs have long histories as safe healers—in Asia, for example, angelica has long been used to treat arthritis. But to claim this on the package, the manufacturer would have to get the FDA to approve angelica as a new drug—a lengthy process that costs more than $200 million, experts estimate.

Since natural substances such as herbs cannot be patented, it would never be profitable to go through the approval process, says Daniel B. Mowrey, Ph.D., director of the American Phytotherapy Research Laboratory in Salt Lake City, Utah, and author of *The Scientific Validation of Herbal Medicine*. This is also the reason that big drug companies have little interest in exploring even the most promising herbal remedies.

To sidestep the problem of FDA regulation, herb purveyors have simply sold their products as food supplements, without therapeutic claims. Unfortunately, that leaves the consumer without a clue as to a product's uses or possible risks and with no assurance of its potency or quality, says Varro E. Tyler, Ph.D., professor of pharmacognosy at Purdue University School of Pharmacy in West Lafayette, Indiana, and author of *The Honest Herbal*. According to some studies of expensive herbal products, he says, "consumers have less than a 50 percent chance of actually getting what the label says they're buying."

As Dr. Farnsworth warns, "When it comes to herbal products, it's 'buyer beware.'"

Out of the Maze

Given this confusion, here are a few ways to help you pick safely from nature's garden of healing plants.

Educate yourself. Read up on herbs, but be skeptical. Today's self-styled herbalists seldom have a good background in chemistry and botany, says Dr. Tyler, and many rely on outdated or inaccurate information. As long as it's not part of the labeling, they may make outrageous claims for an herb's healing powers, he says. Look for experts with credentials in medicine or pharmacognosy—the science of discovering medicinal products in nature.

Don't play doctor. Never diagnose yourself or use any "alternative" therapy instead of a proven med-

Caution: Plants Can Be Dangerous

Not all herbal products are safe. Although the following is not a complete list of unsafe plants, those listed here deserve special attention.

The herbs in this list are dangerous; do not use as remedies.

Borage	Harmful in large doses; may cause liver damage and cancer
Broom	Toxic; powerful laxative
Chapparal	May cause illness; banned in the U.S.
Coltsfoot	May cause cancer
Comfrey	May cause liver damage and cancer (but not through external use)
Foxglove	Potent heart toxin
Pennyroyal	The essential oil may cause convulsions in large doses; possibly harmful to pregnant women
Pokeweed	Poisonous
Rue	Dangerous to pregnant women
Sassafras	May cause cancer
Sweet woodruff	Large doses may cause dizziness and vomiting

These herbs are potentially dangerous; use with caution.

Aloe	Used internally, a powerful laxative
Goldenseal	Poisonous in large doses
Juniper	Should not be used by pregnant women or people with kidney disease
Licorice	Excessive amounts may cause fluid retention and high blood pressure

ical treatment without telling your doctor first, says Alan R. Gaby, M.D., a Baltimore physician who practices nutritional and natural medicine and is president of the American Holistic Medical Association. "In some cases, you can use herbs and other natural treatments as a substitute for conventional medicine," he says, "but there are also curative treatments you'll miss if you don't go for a checkup." Unless you're absolutely sure what's wrong, he advises, don't try to self-medicate.

If you wish to try herbal remedies, says Dr. Farnsworth, use them for conditions that you know are not serious and will eventually clear up by themselves—for example, colds or minor arthritis pain. If a chronic condition persists or gets worse, see your doctor.

And when it comes to such life-threatening diseases as cancer or AIDS, beware of peddlers or practitioners who prey on desperate people, says Dr. Beutler. If a so-called cure sounds too good to be true, it probably is.

Don't presume that "natural" equals "safe." According to Dr. Farnsworth, "People often presume that just because an herb is a plant, it's safe to use. That's not necessarily true. Some of the most virulent toxins known come from plants."

Many herbs have been used by thousands of people for hundreds of years with virtually no ill effects and possibly much benefit. But occasionally there are reports of herbal remedies causing sickness or even a rare death. Often, says Dr. Farnsworth, the herbs may have been misidentified or adulterated with other plants or toxic substances. He advises buying herbs and herbal products only from reputable growers and manufacturers.

Start low and go slow. If you try a new herbal product, start with the lowest dose, and if you experience no benefit after a week or so, increase it gradually, recommends Dr. Farnsworth. Don't take more than the recommended amount, however, and don't take high doses of any remedy for months or years unless the long-term effects have been well studied. For most herbs, he adds, the active ingredients and long-term effects are poorly understood or unknown.

If you feel worse after taking an herbal remedy, stop taking it. Allergies or other adverse reactions to any plant substance are always a possibility. If an herb disagrees with you or if you develop any new symptoms after taking it, discontinue use.

Avoid herbal remedies if you are pregnant, nursing or taking other medication. Little is known about the effects of herbs or their active ingredients on an unborn child or on a baby through breast milk. It's best to err on the side of caution, says Dr. Farnsworth. He also advises against mixing herbal remedies with prescription or over-the-counter drugs—an herb may make the action of another medication weaker or stronger.

How to Use Herbs

It's easy to take aspirin: Just read the label, which says something like "take every four hours." But what about herbs? Whether you grow your own herbs or buy them from a health food store, you're faced with a challenge. Sometimes—as with many herbal teas—there's a label to help you. But some herbs come in many forms. Echinacea, for example, can be purchased in the form of capsules, tinctures or tea; alone or combined with other herbs; in a concentrated extract or in a prepara-

9

Buying Herbal Products

Using herbs is simple. You just pick some up in your local health food store and . . . Whoa! Stop! Halt! The fantasy of the no-fuss, no-trouble use of herbs is all too frequently just that—a fantasy. You may do quite well buying bulk herbs locally, but the fact of the matter is that the quality of commercially sold herbs varies widely.

Dried herbs may lose their potency quickly if not stored properly. More expensive herbs are often adulterated or otherwise tampered with. Even packaged products are not sacrosanct. Investigators have found, for example, that often products labeled "ginseng" contain either an inexpensive substitute or none whatsoever of the costly herb.

Herbal products are not subject to government regulation for quality, potency or authenticity. What's a person who wants to use herbs to do?

In general, beware of products that are accompanied by extravagant health claims or that are exorbitantly expensive. Herbal experts advise purchasing herbs only from reputable companies with a name and reputation to protect.

tion made from the fresh roots and flowers. Which one do you choose?

Here again, there are no easy answers. Some herbalists believe that products made from the whole plant are superior to preparations containing only the "active ingredients." Mother Nature, they reason, knows best what subtle combination of compounds will deliver

The following firms are well-known suppliers to naturopathic physicians. All sell directly to the public, either through retailers such as health food stores or by mail order.

Cardiovascular Research/
   Ecological Formulas
c/o L&H Vitamins
37-10 Crescent Street
Long Island City, NY
   11101

Eclectic Institute
14385 S.E. Lusted Road
Sandy, OR 97055

Herb and Spice Collection
3021 78th Street
P.O. Box 118
Norway, IA 52318-0118

Herb Pharm
Box 116
Williams, OR 97544

Nature's Herb Company
1010 46th Street
Emeryville, CA 94608

Nature's Way
P.O. Box 4000
Springville, UT 84663

Penn Herb Company
603 North 2nd Street
Philadelphia, PA 19123

Pharmacists Nutrition
   Center
9775 SW Commerce
   Circle, Suite CS
Portland, OR 97070

the most benefits with the fewest side effects. Other herbalists prefer standardized extracts.

Herbalism remains an inexact science. A plant's therapeutic activity in the human body may vary with its time of harvest, the methods of storage and cultivation, the dosage and what else is going on in the body. Like the medicine men and wise women of old,

today's herb user must rely to a great extent on trial
and error to discover which products seem to work
best.

"People often ask about the right dose, but we
may not need to get that technical," says Steven
Dentali, Ph.D., quality assurance director and natural
products chemist for Trout Lake Farm and Flora Laboratories in Trout Lake, Washington, and a private
herbal consultant. "Take an herb with a history of safe
use, for a self-limiting condition, and find out what it
does for you."

Back to the Future

Herbal medicine has become big business in the
United States, although it is still just a sprout compared
to the giant pharmaceutical industry. This herbal re-
naissance has grown out of consumer demand: People
are beginning to try herbs, and they like what they are
finding.

Don't look for herbs to take the place of wonder drugs any time soon. But some scientists, like Dr. Farnsworth, see real hope for herbs to help bolster the body's immune response and ease chronic conditions like asthma and arthritis.

And then there's all that research that's looking into the potential of plant-derived substances as cancer treatments. "I can't say there's another taxol ready to emerge from the research pipeline, but we're encouraged. We see some very interesting things ahead," says Dr. Beutler.

More research is, in fact, the key to unlocking the age-old potential of healing herbs for treating a wide variety of human ills. Herb enthusiasts are heartened, for example, by the fact that the prestigious National Institutes of Health in 1991 established an Office of Alternative Medicine to evaluate the scientific merit of herbalism and other nonstandard healing methods. And a small but growing number of medical doctors are already combining so-called alternative techniques such as herbalism and acupuncture with standard medical practice.

In the end, though, ordinary people—not doctors and scientists—are the ones bringing nature and medicine together again. "Herbs are people medicine," says Dr. Dentali. And if people use them appropriately, he says, they can be effective medicine indeed, readily available to anyone.

"Herbs are a reminder that our lives depend absolutely on plants. Grow them, use them, enjoy them," he says.

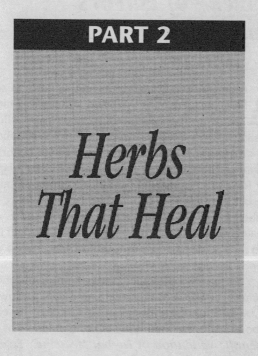

PART 2

Herbs That Heal

Allspice

A Blend of Flavors and Benefits

Allspice owes its name to its unique flavor: a zesty blend of cinnamon, pepper, juniper and clove. Thanks to its oil, it also has mild but significant healing powers as a digestive aid and topical anesthetic.

Aromatic allspice berries have a long history in Caribbean folk healing. Jamaicans drink hot allspice tea for colds, menstrual cramps and upset stomach. Costa Ricans use it to treat indigestion, flatulence and diabetes. Cubans consider it a refreshing tonic. And Guatemalans apply crushed berries to bruises and joint and muscle pains. Most of these uses have been confirmed by modern science.

"Allspice owes its medicinal actions to eugenol, a chemical constituent of its oil," says Daniel B. Mowrey, Ph.D., director of the American Phytotherapy Research Laboratory in Salt Lake City, Utah, and author of *The Scientific Validation of Herbal Medicine*. "Eugenol promotes digestion by enhancing the activity of the digestive enzyme trypsin. It's also an effective pain reliever and anesthetic."

Dentists use eugenol as a local anesthetic for teeth and gums, and the chemical is an ingredient in the over-the-counter toothache remedies Numzident and Benzodent.

"Allspice oil is not as rich in eugenol as clove oil," says James A. Duke, Ph.D., a botanist retired from the U.S. Department of Agriculture and author of *The CRC Handbook of Medicinal Herbs*. That's why dentists favor clove oil. But allspice oil has similar anesthetic action and may be applied directly to painful teeth as first aid until professional care can be obtained.

Putting the Herb to Work

For toothache, apply allspice oil directly to the tooth, one drop at a time, using a cotton swab. Take care not to swallow it. Powdered allspice adds a warm, rich flavor to foods, but its highly concentrated oil should never be swallowed. As little as one teaspoon can cause nausea, vomiting and even convulsions.

Allspice is on the Food and Drug Administration's list of herbs generally regarded as safe. But in people with sensitive skin, particularly those with eczema, allspice oil may cause inflammation. If inflammation develops, stop using it.

For a medicinal tea, use one to two teaspoons of allspice powder per cup of boiling water. Steep for 10 to 20 minutes and strain. Drink up to three cups a day. When using commercial preparations, follow the package directions.

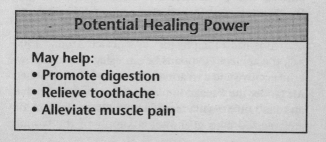

Potential Healing Power

May help:
• Promote digestion
• Relieve toothache
• Alleviate muscle pain

Aloe

Herbal First Aid

As a healing plant, aloe is something of a celebrity. Across America, the spiky plant sits on untold numbers of kitchen windowsills, just waiting. Waiting for what? A spattered bit of grease, a careless moment at the oven, and the inner gel of the aloe leaves gets called into service as a burn salve. Even scientists take advantage of this simple home remedy.

"To treat minor burns, scalds and cuts, I keep a potted aloe on the windowsill of my kitchen," says Daniel B. Mowrey, Ph.D., director of the American Phytotherapy Research Laboratory in Salt Lake City, Utah, and author of *The Scientific Validation of Herbal Medicine*. "Everyone should."

Most household burns and scalds, and many other minor mishaps, occur in the kitchen. With an aloe plant close by, it's easy to snip off one of the thick, fleshy leaves, slit it open and squeeze the clear gel onto the injury. "Aloe gel dries into a natural bandage," Dr. Mowrey explains. "It also promotes healing and helps keep burns from becoming infected."

Aloe has a long history as a healer. Around 1500 B.C., the ancient Egyptians began using aloe as a powerful laxative and a treatment for skin problems. When Alexander the Great conquered Egypt, he learned that an island off Somalia teemed with aloes. He immediately seized it to guarantee a supply of the wound treatment for his troops, while keeping the herb from his enemies. Arab traders carried aloe from Spain to Asia around the sixth century. Traditional Indian Ayurvedic doctors and Chinese physicians quickly adopted it as a laxative and skin treatment. American pioneers used aloe gel to treat wounds, burns, hemorrhoids and rashes.

Scientific validation of aloe's wound-healing power dates from the 1930s, when radiologists noticed that aloe gel scooped straight from the cut leaves of the plant hastened the healing of x-ray burns. Since then, many studies have confirmed the herb's ability to promote healing of cuts, frostbite and first- and second-degree burns.

"Aloe contains allantoin, a substance that speeds wound healing," says Alan R. Gaby, M.D., a Baltimore physician who practices nutritional and natural medicine and is president of the American Holistic Medical Association.

One chemical in this herb—aloe-emodin—"has anti-tumor activity," according to James A. Duke, Ph.D., a botanist retired from the U.S. Department of Agriculture and author of *The CRC Handbook of Medicinal Herbs*. Aloe is not currently used to treat cancer, but one day it might be. And some derivatives of aloe

---

Potential Healing Power

May help:
• Heal burns and scalds
• Relieve sunburn
• Treat minor wounds

---

are also being studied for both anti-AIDS and anti-cancer potential.

Squeeze a Leaf for Relief

Before applying aloe to burns or cuts, wash them thoroughly with soap and water. For minor burns, scalds, sunburns or cuts, select a lower (older) leaf, cut off several inches and slice it lengthwise. Scoop out the gel, apply it liberally to the affected area and allow it to dry. (The injured aloe leaf quickly closes its own wound. Periodic leaf-snipping does not harm the plant.)

Aloe gel is safe for external use by anyone who does not develop an allergic reaction. If your skin shows signs of redness or irritation after using aloe, discontinue use. And if a burn or cut does not heal significantly within two weeks, consult a physician.

Even if you have a brown thumb, you can grow aloes. They need little water and no care other than good drainage and a temperature above 40°F. They prefer sun but tolerate shade, and they don't mind poor soil. Aloes periodically produce offshoots, which may be removed and replanted when they are a few inches tall. Simply uproot or unpot the plant, work the soil gently to separate the offshoot and return the parent plant to its bed or pot.

Angelica

Regaining Popularity as Dang-qui

In the West, Chinese angelica's time came and largely went. But now, after more than a century as a minor healer, this eight-foot plant, once called wild celery, has returned to popularity, thanks to its place of honor in Chinese medicine.

Chinese angelica, also known as *dang-qui* or *tang-kuei*, "is the leading Chinese herb for gynecological health," says Pi-Kwang Tsung, Ph.D., former assistant professor of pathology at the University of Connecticut Medical School in Farmington and currently editor of *The East-West Medical Digest.*

Treatment of gynecological problems is a far cry from angelica's uses in medieval Europe, where peasants made necklaces from the leaves of European angelica (*Angelica archangelica*) to protect their children from illness and witchcraft.

The herb became medically prominent because of an epidemic of bubonic plague in 1665. Legend has it that a monk dreamed an angel told him that wild celery could cure the dread disease. The monk renamed the plant "angelica" in honor of his dream-visitor, and not long afterward, the British Royal College of Physicians incorporated the herb into its official

Potential Healing Power
May help: • **Relieve menstrual discomfort** • **Minimize symptoms of menopause** • **Treat colds and other respiratory problems** • **Prevent arthritis** • **Combat certain cancers**

plague treatment, The King's Excellent Plague Recipe. Despite the recipe's supposed excellence, plague killed tens of thousands, and faith in angelica's healing abilities plummeted.

By the eighteenth century, European herbalists had relegated angelica to the relatively insignificant role of treating minor respiratory complaints, cold symptoms and coughs. These uses appear to be scientifically based. "In German animal studies, the oil in angelica has shown a relaxing effect on the trachea (windpipe)," says Bernie Olin, Pharm.D., editor of *The Lawrence Review of Natural Products,* a St. Louis–based newsletter that summarizes scientific research on medicinal herbs.

Women's Healer from China

Asian physicians maintain that Chinese angelica *(A. sinensis)* is considerably more valuable than the European variety. For thousands of years, Chinese and traditional Indian Ayurvedic physicians have prescribed it as *the* tonic for gynecological problems.

"Studies show that dang-qui increases red blood

22

cell counts," Dr. Tsung explains. "That's why Chinese physicians give it to women who have just given birth. Childbirth involves blood loss, and dang-qui helps the body replace lost red blood cells."

Angelica also helps relax the uterus, and combined with other Chinese herbs it can stimulate secretion of the female sex hormone estrogen. Low estrogen levels can cause menstrual problems and are responsible for many menopausal complaints. Dang-qui helps minimize them.

But Chinese angelica is not just for women, according to Dr. Tsung. Dang-qui's ability to boost the production of red blood cells explains why it is used for treating weakness and fatigue in both men and women. Red blood cells carry oxygen to the tissues. As red blood cells proliferate, oxygenation of the blood increases, enabling the body to function more efficiently.

Also, "an immune-stimulating substance has been identified in dang-qui," Dr. Tsung says, "which can help both men and women stay healthy." In particular, he says, it may help prevent chronic diseases such as cancer and arthritis.

On the other hand, Varro E. Tyler, Ph.D., professor of pharmacognosy at Purdue University School of Pharmacy in West Lafayette, Indiana, and author of *The Honest Herbal,* remains skeptical of claims for dang-qui: "Chinese research is not always as rigorous as it ought to be, so I don't consider this herb to have proven benefit."

Calling on the Angel

Herbal experts recommend using European angelica for respiratory complaints and dang-qui for gyneco-

23

logical health and stimulating the immune system. To make a medicinal tea, use one teaspoon of crushed root per cup of boiling water. Steep for 10 to 20 minutes.

Angelica has a fragrant aroma and a warm, vaguely sweet taste reminiscent of juniper, followed by a bitter aftertaste. When using a commercial preparation, follow package directions.

Anise

Licorice-Flavored Gas Reliever

Anise is a flavor appreciated by connoisseurs of fine liquors around the world—the Greeks have their ouzo and the French their pastis. But aside from its use as a flavoring agent, aniseed is valued for other reasons as well.

As far back as the days of the ancient Greeks and Romans, the licorice-flavored herb was used for various medicinal purposes, including freshening the breath, relieving gas, promoting milk production in nursing mothers and helping expel excess phlegm.

And there just may be something to a few of these ancient claims. Today, herb experts particularly tout anise's ability as a digestive aid and gas reliever. Anise is quite safe—anyone who has an upset stomach or gas can give it a try, according to James A. Duke, Ph.D., a botanist retired from the U.S. Department of Agriculture and author of *The CRC Handbook of Medicinal Herbs*.

Calming Colic

Anise can also be effective in relieving colic in infants, says Dr. Duke. "People tend to use dill and fennel more, but they all have the same properties," he says.

To make anise tea to calm the stomach or relieve gas, crush one teaspoon of aniseed and mix it in one cup of boiling water. Steep for 10 to 20 minutes. Drink up to three cups a day. For additional digestive relief, Dr. Duke recommends adding fresh or dried peppermint leaf. You can also chew a handful of the seeds to freshen your breath.

To give anise tea to an infant, dilute ½ cup of tea with ½ cup of water. And make sure you allow it to cool sufficiently.

Potential Healing Power

May help:
• Settle upset stomach
• Relieve gas
• Soothe colic

Astragalus

Chinese Immune System Booster

Astragalus, used as a tonic in traditional Chinese medicine since antiquity, is now finding its way to the shelves of American health food stores. Also called milk vetch, astragalus is a member of the legume, or bean, family. The sweet-tasting roots, which are the parts used medicinally, are black with a pale yellow core. In Chinese, the herb is called *Huang-qi,* or "yellow leader." Researchers in both the United States and China have found clues that it may well live up to its 2,000-year-old reputation as an immune system booster.

"Astragalus is one of the most commonly used herbs in all of Chinese medicine," according to Subhuti Dharmananda, Ph.D., director of the Institute for Traditional Medicine in Portland, Oregon. Chinese herbalists prescribe it to build up the vital energy, or *qi* (pronounced *key*), of a weakened person, he explains, and include it in many combination remedies to promote the action of other herbs. It's used to promote urination, speed healing of burns and abscesses and generally bolster the body's resistance to disease.

Chinese healers also use astragalus to treat the common cold, arthritis, weakness, diarrhea, asthma and nervousness. Sometimes they pan-roast the roots in honey or use them as an ingredient in soup.

Cancer Therapy Helper

In Chinese hospitals, astragalus is used to help people with cancer recover from the immune system wipeout caused by chemotherapy.

In research conducted at the M. D. Anderson Cancer Center in Houston, a team of Chinese and American scientists studied the effects of compounds taken from astragalus roots on immune system cells taken from people with cancer and AIDS. The results: The researchers noted an increase in the functioning of T-cells, which are key fighters in the body's immune defense network. These were test-tube studies, though, and there's no proof yet that people with cancer who take astragalus preparations will benefit.

Cancer isn't the only ill for which astragalus may hold promise. In Shanghai, doctors have shown that compounds from the root can protect heart cells from damage caused by the Coxsackie B virus, which can scar the hearts of both adults and infants. In one experiment, people suffering from this viral infection not

Potential Healing Power
May help: • **Bolster immunity**   • **Heal burns and abscesses**   • **Offset adverse effects of cancer therapy**   • **Protect the heart against viral damage**

only improved but showed enhanced resistance to the common cold.

Putting Astragalus to Work

Astragalus preparations are available at many health food stores in the form of capsules, teas and tinctures. To prepare them, simply follow the directions on the package. The herb has not been reported to cause dangerous side effects, according to Dr. Dharmananda, but some people report loose stools or abdominal bloating. If you experience any unpleasant symptoms, cut back your dose or discontinue use.

An important note: There are many flowering plants in the astragalus family, including native American species that are toxic when eaten by cattle. (Ranchers call the plant locoweed because of its effect on their herds' behavior.) The particular herb known as astragalus in Chinese medicine is a species called *Astragalus membranaceus.*

For the maximum benefit from astragalus, Dr. Dharmananda recommends consulting a Chinese herbalist or other practitioner trained in traditional Chinese medicine. Like other Chinese herbs, "yellow leader" is often prescribed with a complex blend of other herbs and foods for maximum effect.

Astragalus itself is not a cancer cure; as with any traditional therapy, don't add it to a treatment regimen without discussing it with your doctor.

Balm

All-Purpose Soother

Stomach comforter, blues banisher, herpes fighter, even bug repellent: The reputed uses of balm are so varied that it's no wonder this lemon-scented herb has been nicknamed "cure-all."

Although its therapeutic usefulness is little known in this country, balm (sometimes referred to as lemon balm but officially called *Melissa officinalis*) is widely used and highly valued by legitimate herbal practitioners in Western Europe.

The leaves of this pungent member of the mint family have been used medicinally for some 2,000 years. The eleventh-century Arab physician Avicenna believed it "causeth the mind and heart to become merry" and recommended it to dispel melancholy.

Balm was considered a must-have plant for Elizabethan herb gardens, and over the centuries it seems to have been a popular home remedy for a host of common ailments. "Let a syrup made with the juice of it and sugar . . . be kept in every gentlewoman's house to relieve the weak stomachs and sick bodies of their poor sickly neighbours," wrote English physician Nicholas Culpeper in *The Complete Herbal* of 1653.

Modern research has suggested that there may be some truth to some, if not all, of these folk uses.

Potential Healing Power

May help:
- Heal minor wounds
- Ease indigestion
- Relieve menstrual cramps
- Treat cold sores
- Relax nerves
- Aid sleep
- Repel insects

There's no proof that balm makes you merry, but various small-scale laboratory studies in Germany have demonstrated that balm leaves contain compounds with sedative, digestive and anti-spasmodic effects, says Varro E. Tyler, Ph.D., professor of pharmacognosy at Purdue University School of Pharmacy in West Lafayette, Indiana, and author of *The Honest Herbal*. Culpeper's crude recipe, then, may indeed help relieve tummy troubles.

Help for Herpes?

Recent research has shown another use for balm that the Elizabethans never dreamed of: battling herpes simplex, the virus that causes cold sores. "That's pretty well documented," says Dr. Tyler, adding that a cream containing highly concentrated balm compounds, sold in Europe but unavailable in the United States, has been shown to speed the healing of herpes lesions and lengthen the time between outbreaks.

Can you heal herpes by drinking balm tea? Don't bet on it. "You can't kill the herpes virus by taking it internally," says Norman R. Farnsworth, Ph.D., director of the Program for Collaborative Research in the Pharmaceutical Sciences at the University of Illinois at Chicago. "The studies showing antiviral activity are probably due to the tannins in balm; applied externally, they may act as an astringent and kill some surface viruses." Even applied externally, balm leaves or home brews probably aren't strong enough to be effective, says Dr. Tyler: "The tea would contain the tannins, but not in the same concentration as a commercial preparation."

Balm causes no documented safety problems, although it has been shown to inhibit certain thyroid hormones. For this reason, people with Graves' disease or other thyroid-related problems should use this herb cautiously, if at all.

Balm has another potential virtue: While bees may love it, mosquitoes reportedly hate it.

Using Balm

Modern herbalists recommend a balm tea made from fresh or dried leaves to calm the nerves, aid sleep, ease menstrual cramps and reduce fever. Use about two teaspoons of chopped leaves (preferably fresh, not dried) to one cup of boiling water. Steep 10 to 20 minutes and drink while hot. Balm tincture is another option, with the usual dose being a teaspoon or less as needed.

Balm leaves are a fragrant and soothing addition to herbal baths or pillows. You can also apply a poultice of the crushed leaves to soothe insect bites and stings and help heal wounds, according to Dr. Farnsworth. Balm's properties as an insect repellent are unproven, but you might try rubbing balm oil, or the pleasantly scented leaves themselves, over your skin on a summer night, just in case.

Black Haw

Menstrual Pain Reliever

In the nineteenth century, women with menstrual cramps couldn't reach into a medicine cabinet for Midol. Instead they drank a tea made from black haw bark. The "uterine tonic," first written about in 1857, was reputed to relieve menstrual pain, prevent miscarriage and ease the pain that follows childbirth.

Women have been using it ever since to relieve menstrual cramps. "I used to work in a drugstore in Massachusetts when I was in college, and a product called Hayden's Viburnum Compound was sold," recalls Norman R. Farnsworth, Ph.D., director of the Program for Collaborative Research in the Pharmaceutical Sciences at the University of Illinois at Chicago. "It was the worst-smelling and -tasting thing. But women would come in and swear that when they had menstrual cramps, it worked." (*Viburnum prunifolium* is the scientific name for the herb.)

Can women today turn to black haw bark tea as an alternative to their over-the-counter medications? It may, in fact, be helpful.

The bark contains substances that appear to affect smooth muscle, says Glenn S. Rothfeld, M.D., clinical instructor in the Department of Community Health at Tufts University School of Medicine in Boston. "These substances have been shown to work actively on the uterus, particularly to relax it," he says.

"I would not encourage women to use black haw or other herbs to prevent miscarriage unless they are under someone's care who has expertise in treating with herbs," says Dr. Rothfeld. But the herb may be used for relieving menstrual cramps, he says. Pregnant women shouldn't take any herb for health or healing without the consent of an obstetrician.

To make a decoction or tea from black haw bark, says Dr. Rothfeld, use one ounce of herb to a pint of freshly boiled distilled water. Steep for 10 to 15 minutes and strain. Drink one cup two to three times a day to relieve cramping, he says.

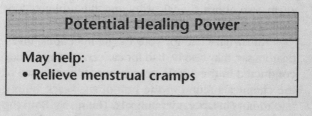

Potential Healing Power

May help:
• **Relieve menstrual cramps**

Black Walnut

Fungus Terminator

Expert gardeners know better than to plant under the black walnut tree.

"Have you ever seen what grows under a black walnut tree? Nothing. There's a reason for that: It contains a chemical that kills anything that it comes in contact with," says Christopher W. W. Beecher, Ph.D., associate professor of pharmacognosy in the Department of Medicinal Chemistry and Pharmacognosy at the University of Illinois at Chicago.

Some American Indian tribes apparently recognized black walnut bark's destructive power and turned it against conditions like ringworm, a fungal skin infection. "For something like ringworm, a topical application of this chemical is going to go right in there and bind to the infected cells. And that should be the end of the fungus," says Dr. Beecher. Black walnut's active component may also be effective against stubborn fungal problems like athlete's foot and jock itch.

And what's bad for your fungal infections, investigators say, may also be bad for cancer. During a study conducted in the 1960s, researchers injected two of the chemicals found in the hull of the black walnut into tumors in laboratory animals. The result: Both the size and the weight of the tumors decreased dramatically. Researchers investigating the same effect obtained a German patent in 1990 for this anti-cancer treatment.

Black walnut fruit, on the other hand, also seems to show promise in the fight against deadly disease. Although much more research needs to be done, preliminary studies conducted during the 1960s revealed that large doses of the chemicals in the nut could help lower blood pressure. And perhaps even different walnuts don't fall too far from the tree: More recent studies of the English walnut have documented its effectiveness in helping lower cholesterol as part of a heart-healthy diet.

Kiss Fungus Good-Bye

If you'd like to try black walnut's potent fungus-fighting power for yourself, you can purchase a liquid extract at many health food stores. Follow the package instructions before applying it to your skin.

Black walnut extract capsules are also available at health food stores, but, in view of their toxicity, Dr. Beecher suggests consulting a health professional before using them.

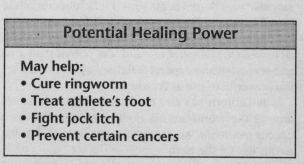

Potential Healing Power
May help: • Cure ringworm • Treat athlete's foot • Fight jock itch • Prevent certain cancers

Buckthorn

Possible Cancer Treatment

Buckthorn became popular in European herbal medicine about 1,000 years ago. At the time, little was known about the body. Doctors believed the key to curing disease lay in purging "foul humours." Not surprisingly, strong laxatives were prescribed for dozens of ailments. Buckthorn was a favorite because it produced reliable results, although it sometimes caused severe gastrointestinal irritation and cramping when people took too much.

Buckthorn's laxative action is the result of chemicals in the plant called anthraquinones. They stimulate the colonic muscle contractions we experience as "the urge." Several other laxative herbs—aloe, cascara sagrada and senna—also contain anthraquinones.

"Buckthorn is about as powerful as cascara sagrada," says Daniel B. Mowrey, Ph.D., director of the American Phytotherapy Research Laboratory in Salt Lake City, Utah, and author of *The Scientific Validation of Herbal Medicine*, "and less potent than aloe and senna." (Some experts feel that aloe and senna are too powerful to use as laxatives.)

Buckthorn has also been used fairly extensively around the world among traditional herbalists as a cancer treatment. And there is apparently something to this use for the herb.

"Buckthorn has shown some anti-tumor action,"

says James A. Duke, Ph.D., a botanist retired from the U.S. Department of Agriculture and author of *The CRC Handbook of Medicinal Herbs*. "It deserves more research."

Harnessing Powerful Laxative Action

In Germany, where herbal healing is more mainstream than it is in the United States, some physicians prescribe a laxative tea containing ½ teaspoon each of buckthorn, fennel seed and chamomile flowers (fennel and chamomile soothe the stomach) per cup of boiling water, steeped for ten minutes. If you try this, drink no more than one cup. It's best to take it before bed.

If you gather your own buckthorn, make sure it has been dried thoroughly before you use it as a laxative. Poorly dried buckthorn can cause vomiting, severe abdominal pain and violent diarrhea.

If you're constipated, you should consider anthraquinone laxatives only as a last resort. Doctors recommend eating a high-fiber diet and getting more exercise as the first line of treatment for constipation. If that doesn't work, the next thing to try, they say, is a bulk-forming laxative, such as psyllium (Metamucil). Only after you've given all these a shot should you move on to an anthraquinone laxative such as buckthorn.

Potential Healing Power

May help:
- Relieve constipation
- Treat certain cancers

Buckthorn should not be used by those with chronic gastrointestinal problems such as ulcers, colitis or hemorrhoids. Pregnant women should also avoid it.

Buckthorn should never be used for more than two weeks, because over time it can cause "lazy bowel syndrome," an inability to move stool without chemical stimulation.

Buckthorn is still a long way from being an accepted cancer treatment. If you have cancer and would like to try this herb in addition to standard therapy, discuss it with your physician.

Burdock

The Tenacious Tonic

Burdock's name is a combination of *bur*, for its spiked seed covers, or burrs, that grab onto anything that touches them, and *dock*, Old English for "plant." Many scientists dismiss burdock as useless, but like its seeds, its reputation clings tenaciously as an herbal healing agent because of its subtle tonic benefits and its intriguing potential as a treatment for cancer.

Throughout history, burdock has been recommended for an astonishing number of illnesses. Ancient Chinese physicians used it to treat colds, coughs, tonsillitis, measles, skin infections and snakebite. Traditional European and American herbalists and homeopaths prescribed it for colds, arthritis, gout, stomach problems, fever, canker sores, leprosy, boils, gonorrhea, ringworm and infertility. They also considered it an excellent diuretic and prescribed it for urinary tract infections, kidney problems and painful urination.

Many of these traditional recommendations still echo through contemporary herb guides. But several herb experts scoff at burdock. Among them is Bernie Olin, Pharm.D., editor of *The Lawrence Review of Natural Products,* a St. Louis–based newsletter that summarizes scientific research on medicinal herbs. Some therapeutic activity has been associated with burdock, he notes, "but there is little evidence to suggest that it is useful in the treatment of any human disease."

True, burdock is not powerfully therapeutic, but Daniel B. Mowrey, Ph.D., director of the American Phytotherapy Research Laboratory in Salt Lake City, Utah, and author of *The Scientific Validation of Herbal Medicine,* insists that it deserves its enduring place in herbal healing because of its value as a tonic—a subtle strengthener with cumulatively helpful effects.

"Burdock's action is mild but real," Dr. Mowrey explains. "It has antibacterial and antiviral powers, and

---

Potential Healing Power

May help:
• Treat certain cancers
• Prevent diabetes

it reduces blood sugar, which helps prevent diabetes. I recommend using a little every day. And when you're ill, use it in addition to standard therapies."

A Potential Cancer Fighter

And after all is said and done, burdock may one day prove valuable as a cancer fighter. Burdock's use against cancer goes way back. The twelfth-century German abbess and herbalist Hildegard of Bingen used burdock to treat cancerous tumors, and down through the centuries it has been used as a tumor treatment in Russia, China, India and the Americas. In the United States, it was an ingredient in the popular but highly controversial Hoxsey Cancer Formula, an alternative therapy marketed from the 1930s to the 1950s by ex-coal-miner Harry Hoxsey.

"Five good foreign studies show intriguing anti-tumor or anti-mutation activity," says Dr. Mowrey. (Most substances that cause genetic mutations also cause cancer.) "Recently," says James A. Duke, Ph.D., a botanist retired from the U.S. Department of Agriculture and author of *The CRC Handbook of Medicinal Herbs*, "the National Cancer Institute became interested in burdock as part of its Designer Foods Program, an effort to use biotechnology to introduce cancer-preventive chemicals into common food crops."

To brew a pleasantly sweet-tasting tonic tea, boil one teaspoon of crushed, dried burdock root in three cups of water for 30 minutes. Drink up to three cups a day. Dr. Duke enjoys eating a soup made from the leaf stalks of fresh burdock, which resemble celery when cooked and taste even better, he says.

When using commercial preparations, follow the package directions.

Of course, cancer requires professional care. If you're being treated for cancer and would like to try burdock in addition to standard therapies, discuss it with your physician.

The Toxicology of Botanical Medicines identifies burdock as a uterine stimulant. Pregnant women should not use it.

Butcher's Broom

Sweep Away Circulatory Problems

Herbal medicine has no shortage of plants called broom. In addition to butcher's broom, there is broom, dyer's broom, Spanish broom and corn broom, among others. They all have tough stems and rigid leaves that make them useful for sweeping. They also are often confused with one another. To prevent mix-ups, it's a good idea to learn the Latin name for butcher's broom—*Ruscus aculeatus.*

Butcher's broom is closely related to asparagus, and its young shoots can be prepared and eaten just like the familiar vegetable. If the shoots go unharvested, this herb becomes a low-growing evergreen shrub.

Ancient Greek physicians recommended butch-

Potential Healing Power

May help:
• Relieve hemorrhoids
• Treat leg vein problems

er's broom as a laxative and diuretic, but this herb did not become widely used in healing until the 1950s, when French scientists isolated two chemicals from butcher's broom rhizomes (underground stems). These chemicals have therapeutic value in that they cause blood vessels to narrow and help reduce inflammation.

Following this research, herbalists immediately began recommending butcher's broom for treatment of hemorrhoids, which result from distended veins in the anal area. The final word isn't in yet on whether or not it works. Over time, however, anecdotal reports accumulated that the herb helped treat a lower-leg condition called venous insufficiency or chronic phlebopathy, meaning that the veins there don't function properly, causing swelling, itching, tingling, cramping and a feeling of heaviness.

Studies of butcher's broom for leg vein problems have produced intriguing results. A scientifically rigorous 1988 study showed that a combination of butcher's broom, vitamin C and another chemical found in citrus fruits improved symptoms. "The swelling, itching and tingling improved greatly," says Bernie Olin, Pharm.D., editor of *The Lawrence Review of Natural Products*, a St. Louis–based newsletter that summarizes scientific research on medicinal herbs.

Cramping and heaviness were also relieved to a small extent.

Brewing Up the Broom

Although questions remain about this herb's effectiveness, Daniel B. Mowrey, Ph.D., director of the American Phytotherapy Research Laboratory in Salt Lake City, Utah, and author of *The Scientific Validation of Herbal Medicine*, recommends it for venous insufficiency. "Just make sure you use a guaranteed potency extract with 10 percent total saponins (the active elements in butcher's broom). Several herb companies market them through health food stores," he says. When using a commercial preparation, follow the package directions.

To make a less potent medicinal tea, use two to four teaspoons of twigs or one to two teaspoons of fresh rhizome per cup of boiling water. Steep 10 to 20 minutes. Drink up to three cups a day.

Taking butcher's broom requires some caution. If this herb does indeed constrict the leg veins, it might also raise blood pressure, which may increase the risk of heart attack and stroke. Circulatory problems require professional care. Before using butcher's broom for swelling or cramping in the legs, consult your physician.

Camphor

Moth Repellent and Muscle Soother

Who'd ever think that the same odoriferous herb that repels wool-eating moths also soothes muscle aches and pains?

It's true. And the herb is camphor, a white crystalline substance that's distilled from the wood and roots of the camphor tree—a large evergreen that grows in Asia, South America, Florida and California—and has a smell akin to turpentine. You may not be as familiar with this particular herb as you think—these days most commercial products said to contain camphor actually contain a synthetic version of it.

Until it was replaced by more effective repellents such as naphthalene, camphor was an insect-banishing blessing. "People would put cakes or pellets of camphor on their closet shelves or between wool blankets or sweaters," explains Varro E. Tyler, Ph.D., professor of pharmacognosy at Purdue University School of Pharmacy in West Lafayette, Indiana, and author of *The Honest Herbal.* The camphor would vaporize, and its pungent fumes would ward off bugs with a taste for cashmere.

Medically, camphor has a long and varied history, although many of its uses have fallen out of favor because of potential toxicity problems. Camphor in alcohol, for example, which was once popular as a "pick-me-up," can actually cause liver damage.

Easing Muscle Aches

External uses for camphor have stood the test of time.

"For years, one of its most popular uses was as a rub-on oil, called camphor liniment, which consisted of cottonseed oil containing enough dissolved camphor to make a strong 20 percent solution," Dr. Tyler explains.

Camphorated oil was banned by the Food and Drug Administration (FDA) in 1980 after reports of poisoning through accidental ingestion and, less commonly, through skin absorption. But topical creams such as Ben-Gay and Aurum Gold Analgesic, containing up to 11 percent camphor, are available and are considered safe by the FDA. These creams produce a sensation of warmth that helps to counter pain. They also increase blood flow to the area to which they are applied, making your skin rosy-pink.

Vicks VapoRub and Vicks VapoSteam also contain camphor, and there is some evidence that inhaling fumes from a vaporizing camphor ointment rubbed on the chest can help to ease coughing.

You can buy cakes of pure camphor—usually by special order—at a pharmacy and make your own camphorated oil. But you may want to think twice be-

Potential Healing Power
May help: • Soothe muscle aches • Relieve coughs

fore experimenting with this potentially harmful substance. "I believe you are much better off simply buying an over-the-counter product that contains camphor in safe amounts than fooling around with it on your own," Dr. Tyler says. "Ingesting amounts as small as a teaspoonful can be fatal."

Cascara Sagrada

Heavy-Duty Laxative

In Spanish, cascara sagrada means "sacred bark," perhaps because this woody shrub has provided blessed relief for more than a few constipated souls. The reddish-brown bark of this herb is harvested, dried, aged and used as a laxative, either as a powder or a liquid extract.

Cascara sagrada's purgative power has earned it a reputation as the world's most widely used laxative and made it the main ingredient in several over-the-counter laxatives.

"The active ingredients in cascara sagrada—anthraquinones—probably act by irritating the intestines to produce wavelike contractions of the muscles of the intestinal wall," explains Norman R. Farnsworth, Ph.D., director of the Program for Collaborative Research in the Pharmaceutical Sciences at the University of Illinois at Chicago. "Most people see results within eight hours."

Even though laxative products containing cascara sagrada are sometimes marketed as "nature's remedy" or "all-natural," or said to "restore bowel tone," they present the same risks as all stimulant laxatives. If you use them on a regular basis, you can develop a condition known as lazy bowel syndrome—you can't go without chemical stimulation! "A bulk laxative, such as psyllium, is a better choice for long-term chronic constipation," Dr. Farnsworth says.

Some anthraquinones, including some of those found in cascara sagrada, have the ability to kill herpes simplex, the virus that causes cold sores, reports Heinz Rosler, Ph.D., associate professor of medicinal chemistry at the University of Maryland School of Pharmacy in Baltimore.

Another ingredient in cascara sagrada—aloe-emodin—has an anti-leukemia action in laboratory animals, lending some support to the herb's traditional use as an alternative cancer treatment. Unfortunately, aloe-emodin is also quite toxic, and scientists say more research is needed before it can be used to treat leukemia.

Use with Caution

Your best bet for taking cascara sagrada safely is to purchase a product that contains this herb as its active in-

---

Potential Healing Power

May help:
• Relieve constipation
• Treat cold sores

---

gredient and to follow the product directions for use, Dr. Farnsworth says. If you are using the bark of this shrub, make sure it has been aged for at least a year before use. As long as the product is labeled "Cascara Sagrada Bark U.S.P.," you can be sure this has been done. Bark that has not been aged correctly contains chemicals that can cause violent diarrhea and severe intestinal cramps.

To make a laxative tea, boil one teaspoon of well-dried bark in three cups of water for 30 minutes. Drink the tea at room temperature, taking one to two cups a day before bed.

Avoid using cascara sagrada if you are pregnant or have ulcers, ulcerative colitis, irritable bowel syndrome, hemorrhoids or other gastrointestinal conditions.

Cayenne (Red Pepper)

The Hottest Healer

The fiery taste and bright red appearance of cayenne pepper make it one of the world's most noticeable spices. Recently, this herb has become as hot in healing as it is on the tongue. Cayenne has proved remarkably effective at relieving certain types of severe, chronic pain. It also aids digestion and may help prevent heart disease.

Cayenne comes from the Caribbean Indian word *kian*. Today Cayenne is the capital of French Guiana. But ironically, only a tiny fraction of the U.S. red pepper supply comes from South America or the Caribbean; most comes from India and Africa. Tabasco (Louisiana pepper), a close cousin of cayenne with all the same health benefits, grows along the Gulf Coast of the United States.

In India, the East Indies, Africa, Mexico and the Caribbean, red pepper enjoys a long history as a stomach-settling digestive aid. "I believe it works," says Varro E. Tyler, Ph.D., professor of pharmacognosy at Purdue University School of Pharmacy in West Lafayette, Indiana, and author of *The Honest Herbal.* Cayenne assists digestion by stimulating the flow of

Potential Healing Power

May help:
• Aid digestion
• Ease muscle pain
• Relieve cluster headaches
• Reduce arthritis pain
• Lower cholesterol
• Fight shingles pain
• Prevent heart disease
• Treat diabetic foot pain

both saliva and stomach secretions. Saliva contains enzymes that begin the breakdown of carbohydrates, and stomach secretions contain acids and other substances that help digest food.

But most Americans doubt the digestive benefits of cayenne, believing instead that the fiery spice can cause ulcers. It doesn't. In one study, researchers used a tiny video camera to examine subjects' stomach linings after both bland meals and meals liberally spiced with jalapeño peppers, another close cousin of cayenne. Their conclusion: There was no difference. Eating highly spiced meals causes no damage whatsoever to the stomach, they reported. However, this finding relates only to people with normal gastrointestinal tracts. "I wouldn't recommend red pepper to anyone with an ulcer," Dr. Tyler says.

What about the burning sensation in your mouth from eating too much red pepper? The best treatment is a glass of milk. The milk protein washes away capsaicin, the chemical in red pepper that's responsible for its heat.

The Heat That Heals

For centuries, herbalists have recommended rubbing red pepper onto sore muscles and joints. Medically, this is known as a counterirritant, a treatment that causes minor superficial discomfort but distracts the person from the more severe, deeper pain. Heet is one brand of capsaicin counterirritant available over the counter.

Recently, however, red pepper has been shown to provide more compelling relief for certain kinds of chronic pain. For reasons still not completely understood, capsaicin interferes with the action of substance

P—a nerve chemical that sends pain messages to the brain.

"Capsaicin has proved so effective at relieving pain that it's the active ingredient in the over-the-counter cream, Zostrix," says James A. Duke, Ph.D., a botanist retired from the U.S. Department of Agriculture and author of The *CRC Handbook of Medicinal Herbs.*

Doctors now recommend Zostrix for arthritis, diabetic foot pain and the pain of shingles. Shingles is an adult disease caused by the same virus that causes chicken pox in children. The virus remains dormant in the body until later in life when, for unknown reasons, it reappears in some people as shingles, causing a rash on one side of the body that progresses from red bumps to blisters to crusty pox resembling chicken pox. In most adults, shingles clears up by itself within a few weeks. But many experience lingering, sometimes severe, pain.

Research suggests that capsaicin can also help relieve the awful pain of cluster headaches. In one study, people who regularly experienced cluster headaches rubbed a capsaicin preparation inside their nostrils and outside their noses on the same side of the head as the headache pain. Within five days, 75 percent reported less pain and fewer headaches. They also reported burning nostrils and runny noses, but these side effects subsided within a week.

Finally, red pepper may help the heart. "It cuts cholesterol levels and reduces the risk of the internal blood clots which trigger heart attack," says Daniel B. Mowrey, Ph.D., director of the American Phytotherapy Research Laboratory in Salt Lake City, Utah, and author of *The Scientific Validation of Herbal Medicine.*

Harnessing Cayenne's Healing Power

Perhaps the most enjoyable way to enjoy cayenne's medicinal benefits is to simply season your food to taste. Even these small amounts of red pepper are therapeutic.

Remember to wash your hands thoroughly after using either cayenne or Zostrix. Cayenne may be kind to your stomach lining, but you definitely don't want to get any in your eyes.

To aid digestion and possibly reduce the risk of heart disease, experts recommend cayenne in capsules, which are available from most herbal suppliers. Follow the directions on the package.

Celery Seed

A Health-Giving Spice

Celery seed adds a distinctive bite to sauerkraut, a fine-edged sharpness to coleslaw and a tangy zip to soups, stews and salad dressings.

Yet along with its refreshing flavor, scientists have found that celery seed may also be adding protection against cancer, high blood pressure and high cholesterol.

In a study for the National Cancer Institute, Luke Lam, Ph.D., and his colleagues at LKT Laboratories in St. Paul, Minnesota, have been analyzing the chemical constituents of celery seed oil and their effect on living beings.

"We isolated five compounds of interest," says Dr. Lam, who was formerly a researcher at the University of Minnesota. "Then we took three of those compounds and looked for their ability to prevent tumor formation in animals."

The result? "The compound sedanolide was the most active," says Dr. Lam. It and a related compound—butyl phthalide—reduced the incidence of tumors in laboratory animals anywhere from 38 to 57 percent. Whether celery can help prevent cancer in people as well as in animals is not yet known.

Studies also suggest that celery seed may give people an edge on another health front: lower blood pressure. So reports William Keller, Ph.D., professor and head of the Division of Medicinal Chemistry and Pharmaceutics at the Northeast Louisiana University School of Pharmacy in Monroe.

In one study at the University of Chicago, laboratory animals given a daily dose of butyl phthalide experienced a 12 percent reduction in their systolic (the top number) blood pressure over a four-week period.

What's more, laboratory studies also indicate that butyl phthalide may help reduce high cholesterol.

Potential Healing Power

May help:
• Prevent certain cancers
• Regulate blood pressure
• Reduce cholesterol

If you'd like to try celery seed for yourself, you can prepare a tea by pouring boiling water over one teaspoon of freshly crushed seeds. Let it steep for 10 to 20 minutes before drinking.

Chamomile

Calming Comfort

Centuries-old folklore holds that the chamomile flower is both an internal and external healer. Recent research suggests that much of this folklore is based on fact. More than just a popular and fragrant tea, chamomile can help quiet an upset stomach, quench the fires of inflammation and bring a restful night's sleep.

The two species of plant, the Roman and German varieties, both belong to the same family as asters and daisies. The secrets of chamomile's healing power lie in a complex blend of substances found in the flowerheads, which resemble miniature daisies and yield an azure-blue volatile oil when distilled. Various compounds in this oil, with names such as chamazulene, bisabolol and flavonoids, are believed to hold the key to the herb's medicinal properties.

Centuries of Use

Chamomile is one of those herbs with a reputation for being "good for what ails you." Over 400 years ago, herbalists noted that drinking chamomile tea helped indigestion, and bathing in an infusion of the flowers seemed to relieve strained muscles and aching joints. Wherever the body felt hot, sore or itchy, chamomile has been there to provide gentle relief.

In shampoos and rinses, chamomile is alleged to keep blonde hair at its golden best. The herb is also traditionally recommended for redness, heat or swelling associated with burns, arthritis and sprains. Due to its mildness, it is favored for children's ailments, including colic and teething.

Out of the Blue

Today's herbalists still use chamomile for much the same bouquet of remedies. "Chamomile is a very mild sedative, and it probably relieves itching when applied externally," says Norman R. Farnsworth, Ph.D., director of the Program for Collaborative Research in the Phar-

---

Potential Healing Power

May help:
- Reduce inflammation
- Soothe skin irritation and diaper rash
- Lessen toothache and teething pain
- Ease earache
- Combat indigestion and colic
- Calm nerves
- Lessen cold symptoms
- Relieve menstrual cramps
- Prevent stomach ulcers

---

maceutical Sciences at the University of Illinois at Chicago. "And in the best restaurants all over the world, you can get chamomile tea after a big meal. It seems to relax the stomach."

Moreover, "chamomile is one of the few medicinal plants that still have a prominent role in traditional medicine," says Daniel B. Mowrey, Ph.D., director of the American Phytotherapy Research Laboratory in Salt Lake City, Utah, and author of *The Scientific Validation of Herbal Medicine*. European researchers have found that the essential oil of this tiny daisy has anti-inflammatory, anti-spasmodic and analgesic properties, reports Dr. Mowrey.

Some studies, performed on animals, have shown that substances in chamomile oil or extract help prevent stomach ulcers and soothe burned or irritated skin. The herb's sedative power was also observed in tests on mice, adds Dr. Mowrey—although anyone who has ever curled up with a cup of chamomile tea on a cold afternoon may not need a cageful of calm mice to be convinced. So far, however, there has been no scientific study on whether chamomile-rinsed blondes have more fun.

Rx: Using Chamomile

In Europe, chamomile is an ingredient in dozens of remedies. Some of these are available from American herbal and health food suppliers, reports Dr. Mowrey. They include:

Chamomile tincture. Take 10 to 20 drops in water three or four times a day for nervousness, indigestion and menstrual cramps.

Chamomile lotion. Apply to irritated skin, aching teeth and ears.

Chamomile-containing ointment or cream.
Use for wounds and diaper rash.

Chamomile extract. This is a concentrated essence to be used only as directed. A German study showed that home steam inhalation with chamomile extract eased the sniffly miseries of the common cold; the stronger the infusion, the greater the relief.

Take Tea and See

Of course, the simplest way to take chamomile is in the form of tea. A cup of chamomile tea delivers a much more diluted dose of active ingredients than commercial products like tinctures or extracts. Even strong tea contains only about 10 to 15 percent of the volatile oil contained in the flowers themselves. However, some experts believe that a daily cup of chamomile tea may have healthful benefits over months or years.

If you would like something stronger than what you would get from a typical chamomile tea bag, brew about a tablespoon of flowerheads per cup of water, then sip. When cooled, the solution can also be used as a refreshing rinse for hair and body. You can also make your own body oil by steeping an ounce of flowers in olive oil for several days, then straining the oil.

Allergy Sufferers, Beware

Chamomile is considered one of the safest herbs, even for children and pregnant women. It is drunk daily by many thousands of people around the world with no problem, points out Varro E. Tyler, Ph.D., professor of pharmacognosy at Purdue University School of Pharmacy in West Lafayette, Indiana, and author of *The*

Honest Herbal. But for a few people, he warns, the pollen-rich flowerheads used to brew the tea can provoke an allergic reaction—in rare cases, a serious one, especially if the person is exposed to other allergens at the same time (for example, during hay fever season).

"If you are allergic to ragweed and other members of the daisy and aster family, such as chrysanthemums, you should be cautious about drinking chamomile tea," says Dr. Tyler. Although chamomile is used in some skin-care products, there have been scattered reports of skin irritation after contact with it. If a chamomile-containing product for external use seems to cause or worsen redness or irritation, he advises, discontinue use.

Cilantro and Coriander

Two Herbs in One

Cilantro and coriander are twin herbs that come from the same plant. Cilantro, sometimes called Chinese parsley, refers to the leaves. Coriander is the name for the seeds. Historically, the seeds were more popular, but today both the leaves and seeds are widely used. And both have the same medicinal benefits in helping to soothe digestion and control infection.

Coriander tastes like a warm combination of sage and citrus. Cilantro has a similar but milder taste. The seeds apparently stimulate the imagination as well as the taste buds, because around the eighth century, the mythical Arabian princess Scheherazade described coriander as an aphrodisiac in the stories later collected as *The Thousand and One Arabian Nights*. (Science is so far silent concerning this use for the seeds.)

Coriander was used as a digestive aid for thousands of years from China to Europe. In Egypt, the seeds were found in pharaohs' tombs, presumably to prevent indigestion in the afterlife. While the Hebrews were slaves in Egypt, they adopted coriander. According to the Bible, God fed them manna, which the holy book says was "like coriander." If manna did what coriander does, the Hebrews did not suffer indigestion. "Cilantro/coriander helps settle the stomach," says James A. Duke, Ph.D., a botanist retired from the U.S. Department of Agriculture and author of *The CRC Handbook of Medicinal Herbs*.

The ancient Romans used both the leaves and the

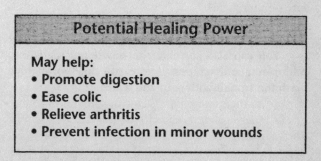

Potential Healing Power

May help:
• Promote digestion
• Ease colic
• Relieve arthritis
• Prevent infection in minor wounds

seeds to preserve meats. And modern Russian researchers have discovered why: The herb is an antioxidant. Antioxidants are chemicals that, among other things, help prevent animal fats from turning rancid. Cilantro and coriander also contain substances that kill meat-spoiling bacteria, fungi and insect larvae. The same microorganisms can cause infections in wounds.

Finally, some studies suggest that cilantro/coriander has anti-inflammatory action, suggesting it might help relieve arthritis.

Try a Spot of Curry

"I've never heard of any problems with cilantro or coriander," says Daniel B. Mowrey, Ph.D., director of the American Phytotherapy Research Laboratory in Salt Lake City, Utah, and author of *The Scientific Validation of Herbal Medicine.* "But some people just don't like it. Quite often when people don't like curry, what they object to is the coriander in it. But curry spices are very healthful."

If you'd rather sip a tea than eat curry, use one teaspoon of dried leaves or crushed seeds (or ½ teaspoon of powdered seeds) per cup of boiling water. Steep for five minutes. Drink up to three cups a day before or after meals.

Weak coriander tea may be given to children under two for colic.

You can also sprinkle the powdered seeds on minor cuts and scrapes. Before you do, thoroughly wash the wound with soap and water.

Cinnamon

Good and Good for You

Hot apple cider tastes flat without a cinnamon stick, and toast, cookies, candies and fruit salads all benefit from a generous sprinkle of cinnamon powder. But cinnamon is more than just a kitchen spice. It's been used medicinally for thousands of years. Modern science has confirmed its value for preventing infection and indigestion and has also discovered a couple of new therapeutic uses for the herb.

Cinnamon comes from the bark of an Asian tree. (The sticks are actually pieces of bark.) Ancient Chinese herbals mention it as early as 2700 B.C., and Chinese herbalists still recommend it for fever, diarrhea and menstrual problems. Cinnamon was an ingredient in ancient Egyptian embalming mixtures. In the Bible, Moses used it in holy anointing oil.

After the fall of Rome, trade between Europe and Asia became difficult, but cinnamon was so prized that it still found its way west. The twelfth-century German abbess and herbalist Hildegard of Bingen recommended it as "the universal spice for sinuses," and to treat colds, flu, cancer and "inner decay and slime," whatever that means.

Boastful Benefits

Several toothpastes are flavored with cinnamon, and for good reason. "Like all the spices used in curries," says

Potential Healing Power

May help:
- Soothe indigestion
- Control blood sugar in people with diabetes
- Prevent stomach ulcers
- Ward off urinary tract infections
- Fight tooth decay and gum disease
- Prevent vaginal yeast infections

Daniel B. Mowrey, Ph.D., director of the American Phytotherapy Research Laboratory in Salt Lake City, Utah, and author of *The Scientific Validation of Herbal Medicine,* "cinnamon is an antiseptic that helps kill the bacteria that cause tooth decay and gum disease." Cinnamon also kills many disease-causing fungi and viruses.

One German study showed it "suppresses completely" the cause of most urinary tract infections (*Escherichia coli* bacteria) and the fungus responsible for vaginal yeast infections (*Candida albicans*).

Like many culinary spices, cinnamon helps soothe the stomach. But a Japanese animal study revealed that it also may help prevent ulcers.

It also appears to help people with diabetes metabolize sugar. In one form of diabetes (Type II, or non-insulin-dependent), the pancreas produces insulin, but the body cannot use it efficiently to break down glucose—the simple sugar that fuels body functions. U.S. Department of Agriculture (USDA) researchers discovered that cinnamon reduces the amount of insulin necessary for glucose metabolism.

Spicing Up Your Health

"One-eighth of a teaspoon of cinnamon triples insulin efficiency," says James A. Duke, Ph.D., a botanist retired from the USDA and author of *The CRC Handbook of Medicinal Herbs*. Dr. Duke suggests that people with Type II diabetes discuss cinnamon's benefits with their doctor.

In foods, simply season to taste. For people with diabetes, ⅛ to ¼ teaspoon of ground cinnamon per meal may help control blood sugar levels.

To brew a stomach-soothing tea, use ½ to ¾ teaspoon of powdered herb per cup of boiling water. Steep 10 to 20 minutes. Drink up to three cups a day.

In powdered form, culinary amounts of cinnamon are nontoxic, although allergic reactions are possible. Cinnamon oil, however, is a different story. On the skin, it may cause redness and burning. Taken internally, it can cause nausea, vomiting and possibly even kidney damage. Don't ingest cinnamon oil.

Clove

Painkilling Preservative

When you were a kid, ham wasn't your favorite food, particularly when Mom studded it with cloves. You tried to pick the little devils out,

Potential Healing Power

May help:
- **Relieve traveler's diarrhea**
- **Calm digestion**
- **Soothe minor wounds and insect bites**
- **Ease toothache**

but one would always slip by and set your entire mouth on fire.

It may have seemed like torture then, but Mom used cloves for a reason. "In addition to providing flavor, cloves are a preservative," says Ara H. Der-Marderosian, Ph.D., professor of pharmacognosy and medicinal chemistry at the Philadelphia College of Pharmacy and Science. "You put cloves in ham and it will last several days longer in the refrigerator."

In addition to their preservative powers, cloves are reputed to have health benefits as well.

Spicy Digestive Relief

In South America, cloves are used to fight digestive disorders; people in Uruguay use tea and liquor made from the spice for relief. The aromatic seeds come from small evergreen trees that grow there, as well as in northeastern Brazil.

The herb's usefulness in combating intestinal problems has yet to be fully tested in humans, but laboratory studies indicate it may be effective. The main component of cloves is eugenol, which has been known for some time to help kill bacteria and viruses, says Gary Elmer, Ph.D., associate professor of medicinal chemistry at the University of Washington School of Pharmacy in Seattle. So drinking clove tea for intestinal problems may be worth a try, he says.

Cloves may even help get your system back on track after travel. Cloves fight a type of bacteria, *Escherichia coli,* which play a role in traveler's diarrhea, says Dr. Elmer. "If you have traveler's diarrhea, you could try clove tea."

The eugenol in cloves also makes the herb effective as an antiseptic and painkiller, says Dr. DerMarderosian. You may have encountered the sweet/hot taste of clove oil in over-the-counter toothache medicines. And while not generally used in the United States, poultices of clove can be used on the skin for cuts and bites. "Indonesians put it on top of wounds, on top of bites, that sort of thing. It has an antiseptic quality," says Dr. DerMarderosian.

Using a poultice of cloves for cuts and bites may be very effective, says Dr. Elmer. Studies show that clove oil can help kill several strains of staphylococcus bacteria and one strain of pseudomonas—organisms that can cause infection in the skin.

Putting Cloves to Work
Clove tea for intestinal problems can be made using one teaspoon of powdered cloves per cup of boiling water. Steep for 10 to 20 minutes before drinking.

To make a poultice for a cut or bite, grind up several cloves, mix them with water and apply the paste to the skin. Cover it with a warm towel.

Coffee

Surprising Benefits from Caffeine

A lthough most people don't think of it as such, coffee is America's most popular herbal beverage. It helps a sleepy nation wake up in the morning. It also has therapeutic value. It can act as a decongestant for colds. It may help prevent asthma attacks. It may boost athletic performance. And it increases the pain-relieving power of aspirin.

Of course, coffee can also cause problems—jitters and insomnia. But despite scare headlines that have linked coffee to many serious diseases, the latest medical review concludes: "Coffee appears to pose no particular threat in most people if consumed in moderation."

Coffee has been around for a long time. Our word *coffee* comes from Caffa, the region of Ethiopia where the fabled beans were first discovered. The beverage we know as coffee emerged around A.D. 1000, when Arabians began roasting and grinding coffee beans and drinking the hot beverage as we do today. Until the seventeenth century, Arabia supplied all the world's coffee through the port of Mocha, which became one of coffee's names. Then the Dutch introduced the plant into Java, and the island quickly became synonymous with coffee.

The medically important constituent of coffee is,

of course, caffeine, but coffee's caffeine content depends on how it's prepared. A cup of instant contains about 60 milligrams of caffeine. Drip or percolated coffee has about 100. A cup of espresso contains about 100 milligrams, too, but this is in a 2½-ounce cup—the traditional serving size for espresso.

Boosting Performance

Coffee is best known as the powerful stimulant that helps people stay awake during night drives and cramming before final exams. It does not, however, help anyone sober up after overindulging in alcohol. In fact, it can upset hung-over stomachs.

Some over-the-counter cold formulas contain caffeine, partly to counteract the sedative effects of the antihistamines they contain. Caffeine may also help open the bronchial tubes, relieving the congestion of colds and flu. Coffee's action as a bronchodilator can also help prevent asthma attacks.

If you take aspirin for pain relief, perhaps you should take it with a cup of coffee. Several studies

---

Potential Healing Power

May help:
- Combat drowsiness
- Temporarily boost athletic performance
- Ease congestion due to colds and flu
- Prevent asthma attacks
- Enhance the pain-relieving effects of aspirin

show that, compared with plain aspirin, the combination of aspirin and caffeine relieves pain significantly better than aspirin alone.

Coffee may also improve physical stamina, according to a report published in the journal *The Physician and Sportsmedicine.* The International Olympic Committee forbids "caffeine loading" and tests urine for illegal amounts. To reach illegal levels, an endurance athlete would have to drink four or five cups in 30 minutes. Athletes who want coffee's benefits without risking disqualification typically drink three or four cups during the hour or two before an event.

How Much Is Too Much?

Caffeine is such an integral part of our culture, we seldom realize how much of a drug it is. The fact is, caffeine is classically addictive. Regular users develop a tolerance and require more to obtain the expected effect. Deprived of caffeine, regular users usually develop withdrawal symptoms, primarily a headache, which can last several days.

Coffee is most notorious for causing insomnia and increasing anxiety, irritability and nervousness. It can also aggravate panic attacks. Coffee increases the secretion of stomach acids and can upset the stomach. Doctors say that people with ulcers or other gastrointestinal conditions should use it cautiously, if at all. Contrary to popular mythology, coffee does not cause ulcers. It can, however, make ulcers worse in people who already have them.

Coffee also raises blood pressure in those who are not accustomed to drinking it. But once java junkies have developed a caffeine tolerance, the body adjusts, and normal consumption no longer affects blood pressure.

But coffee's worst press has concerned its association with heart disease. The subject is extremely controversial, with evidence supporting both sides of the argument. Most studies indicate that coffee can increase cholesterol levels. Oddly, decaffeinated coffee has the same cholesterol-boosting effect as regular, suggesting that caffeine is not the culprit. For reasons that remain a mystery, filtered coffee raises cholesterol less than boiled coffee. If your cholesterol is high, discuss your coffee consumption with your physician.

Independent of coffee's action on cholesterol and blood pressure, it may increase the risk of heart attack. The danger level is more than four cups a day.

There are also reports that coffee aggravates premenstrual syndrome in many women. And coffee has been accused of contributing to infertility, birth defects, gallstones, immune impairment and many forms of cancer. To date, none of these allegations has been proven.

"I'd advise limiting caffeine intake to 250 milligrams a day," says Varro E. Tyler, Ph.D., professor of pharmacognosy at Purdue University School of Pharmacy in West Lafayette, Indiana, and author of *The Honest Herbal.* "That's about two cups of brewed coffee."

"Personally, I drink five or six cups a day," says James A. Duke, Ph.D., a botanist retired from the U.S. Department of Agriculture and author of *The CRC Handbook of Medicinal Herbs.* "But I don't recommend drinking more than two."

Not everyone who quits or cuts back develops withdrawal symptoms, but most people do. The throbbing headache usually begins within 18 to 24 hours and lasts a few days. Constipation is also possible for a day or two.

Dill

From Pickles to Colic

Ever wonder how dill got into dill pickles? Flavor enhancement is only part of the reason. The herb is also a natural preservative, and in the days before refrigeration, vegetables were often pickled in vinegar or brine to preserve them. With dill added, they lasted even longer. Dill also helped settle the stomach, because the herb is a digestive aid.

In fact, the ancient Egyptians, Greeks, Romans and Chinese all used dill to soothe the stomach. The Vikings also appreciated dill's digestive benefits. Our word *dill* comes from the Old Norse *dilla,* meaning "to lull or soothe." During the Middle Ages, dill was used to protect against witchcraft, and throughout history, cooled dill tea, or "dillwater," has been a popular folk remedy for infant colic.

"Dillwater works," says Daniel B. Mowrey, Ph.D., director of the American Phytotherapy Research Laboratory in Salt Lake City, Utah, and author of *The Scientific Validation of Herbal Medicine.* "It's gentle enough for infants."

"For colic, many herbalists recommend a combination of dill and fennel," says James A. Duke, Ph.D., a botanist retired from the U.S. Department of Agriculture and author of *The CRC Handbook of Medicinal Herbs.* "Both herbs contain stomach-soothing oils."

Dill owes its preservative action to its ability to inhibit the growth of several bacteria (staphylococcus, streptococcus, pseudomonas and *Escherichia coli*). This effect suggests that it might help prevent another common early childhood gastrointestinal illness—infectious diarrhea caused by these same microorganisms.

Traditional herbalists also recommended dill for prevention of flatulence, and perhaps there was something to this. The herb has anti-foaming action, suggesting that it might help break up gas bubbles.

How to Do Dill

To brew a stomach-soothing tea, use 2 teaspoons of mashed seeds per cup of boiling water. Steep for ten minutes. Drink up to three cups a day. In a tincture, take ½ to 1 teaspoon up to three times a day.

To treat colic or gas in children under two, give small amounts of a weak tea.

In sensitive individuals, ingesting dill might cause skin rash, but the leaves, seeds and seed oil are generally considered nontoxic. If any skin irritation develops, discontinue use.

Potential Healing Power

May help:
- Improve digestion
- Ease colic
- Fight flatulence
- Prevent infectious diarrhea in children

Echinacea

Nature's Immunity Booster

L ooking at echinacea's reputation through history is like riding a roller coaster. It's up, it's down, it's up again. Before European colonists showed up, the Plains Indians were using this native North American wildflower as a healing herb. The colonists started using it, too, and in the 1870s, a Nebraska doctor popularized it as a "blood purifier" and snakebite remedy.

For years most households in this country kept tincture of echinacea (*ek-i-NAY-see-uh*) on hand as an infection fighter. With the advent of antibiotics, however, the herb fell from favor.

Now, thanks to modern medical science, echinacea is once again receiving favorable attention. Although it's no substitute for antibiotics, this herb holds some promise as an immune system booster after all. In order to reestablish its reputation as a healer, however, this American herb had to do a little traveling. In Germany, extensive research over the past few decades has uncovered a host of infection-fighting properties.

"The herb normalizes the number of white blood cells in the blood and helps them surround and destroy bacteria and viruses," says Daniel B. Mowrey, Ph.D., director of the American Phytotherapy Research Laboratory in Salt Lake City, Utah, and author of *The Scientific Validation of Herbal Medicine*. It also slows the spread of infection to surrounding tissues and helps flush toxins away from infected areas, he says.

In several studies, injections of concentrated compounds derived from echinacea caused people's immune systems to activate macrophages. These germ-gobbling cells are crucial to beating infection, and they may have anti-tumor activity as well. Echinacea may even play a role in curbing the misery of colds and flu. In one study done in Germany, liquid echinacea extract was shown to help ease the symptoms of influenza and speed recovery.

Applied externally as a poultice to wounds, sores and burns, echinacea may also protect against infection and stimulate tissue repair and healing.

Make Sure It's the Real Thing

To battle a cold or the flu, take echinacea at the first sign of symptoms, says Varro E. Tyler, Ph.D., professor of pharmacognosy at Purdue University School of Pharmacy in West Lafayette, Indiana, and author of *The Honest Herbal*. He recommends taking about a teaspoonful of alcohol-based tincture a day to duplicate the effective dose in the German flu study.

A tea made from echinacea provides a tasty but

Potential Healing Power

May help:
- Fight infections
- Reduce symptoms of colds and flu
- Stimulate the immune system
- Heal minor wounds and burns

---

somewhat less potent alternative. To make a tea, pour boiling water over two to three tablespoons of dried, fresh or powdered herb and steep for five minutes. Sip over a period of 30 to 90 minutes and repeat six to eight hours later.

Dr. Tyler warns, however, that the lack of standardization in American herbal products makes it hard to guarantee even an approximate dosage of a particular compound. There have also been reports of echinacea products being adulterated with other herbs. His advice: Purchase herbal products only from well-established, reputable suppliers. Echinacea is generally considered safe, says Dr. Tyler, although an allergic reaction is always a possibility. Discontinue use if you experience any adverse effects.

Ephedra

The World's Original Healer

Ask most people if they've ever heard of Sudafed and they'll say, "Sure, the drugstore decongestant." But ask if they're familiar with the plant it comes from—ephedra—and all they'll say is "Huh?"

Ephedra is one of the world's oldest medicines. Few people who take over-the-counter decongestants containing a component of this herb—pseudoephedrine—have any idea they are participating in an herbal healing tradition that dates back 5,000 years.

The origins of Chinese medicine are lost in legend, but authorities say that Chinese physicians began prescribing Chinese ephedra (*Ephedra sinica*), or *ma huang,* for colds, asthma and hay fever around 3000 B.C.

"Ma huang is the herb for chest congestion and asthma," says Pi-Kwang Tsung, Ph.D., former assistant professor of pathology at the University of Connecticut Medical School in Farmington and currently editor of *The East-West Medical Digest.* "Studies show that its major active constituents are ephedrine and psuedoephedrine."

Unfortunately, not all plants called ephedra have the decongestant benefits of the Chinese variety. American ephedra (*E. nevadensis*), also called Mormon tea, is a pleasant, piney-tasting beverage. "But many studies have shown that it contains no decongestant chemicals," says Bernie Olin, Pharm.D., editor of *The Lawrence Review of Natural Products,* a St. Louis-based newsletter that summarizes scientific research on medicinal herbs.

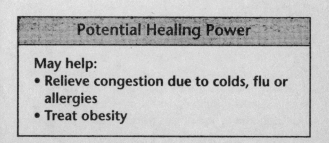

Potential Healing Power

May help:
- Relieve congestion due to colds, flu or allergies
- Treat obesity

Weight Loss, Chinese-Style

The decongestants in Chinese ephedra can also increase basal metabolic rate (BMR)—the speed at which the body burns calories. A few studies have shown that ephedrine-induced increases in BMR can help obese women shed pounds in medically supervised weight-loss programs. The catch is that it only helps those who are seriously obese, not those who want to drop a few extra pounds.

Ephedra can increase heart rate and raise blood pressure, so don't use it if you have high blood pressure, heart disease, diabetes or glaucoma. You should also not take ephedra if you have thyroid problems. In fact, ephedra can be harmful when taken improperly and should not be used by anyone with health problems. If you want to take ephedra or any product containing it, you should discuss it with your doctor.

To brew a medicinal tea, mix one teaspoon of dried ma huang per cup of water, bring it to a boil, then simmer for 10 to 15 minutes. Drink up to two cups a day. In a tincture, take ¼ to 1 teaspoon up to three times a day. When using commercial preparations, follow the package directions.

Eucalyptus

The Australian Antiseptic

I f you've ever used Listerine, Vicks VapoRub, Dristan Nasal Decongestant Spray or Hall's Mentho-Lyptus Cough Suppressants, you're undoubtedly familiar with the unique, refreshing scent of eucalyptus. And if you've ever seen a koala, you've also seen a eucalyptus tree, because its long, scythe-shaped leaves are the sole food source for the cute, furry critter.

Australia's aborigines used eucalyptus to treat fever, cough and asthma—and European settlers quickly adopted it as medicine. For a time, doctors thought eucalyptus could cure malaria, and they called it the Australian fever tree. Alas, that use didn't pan out, but eucalyptus leaf oil does contain a chemical, eucalyptol, that has decongestant and antiseptic action.

"Eucalyptol is a very effective decongestant," says Varro E. Tyler, Ph.D., professor of pharmacognosy at Purdue University School of Pharmacy in West Lafayette, Indiana, and author of *The Honest Herbal.* "It loosens phlegm in the chest, making it easier to cough up. That's why so many decongestants, cough lozenges and chest rubs contain it."

"Eucalyptol also kills several types of bacteria and viruses," says Daniel B. Mowrey, Ph.D., director of the American Phytotherapy Research Laboratory in Salt Lake City, Utah, and author of *The Scientific Validation of Herbal Medicine.* After minor wounds have

Potential Healing Power

May help:
- **Ease congestion**
- **Relieve muscle soreness**
- **Treat minor cuts**

been washed, eucalyptus oil or clean crushed leaves can be applied to help prevent infection.

Recently, a new eucalyptus product, Eucalyptamint, has been promoted as a treatment for muscle soreness. Researchers at the University of California at Irvine tested the ointment and discovered that it increases blood flow to muscle tissue, lending credence to the product's claims.

Using the Australian Healer

To brew a pleasant-tasting medicinal tea, use one to two teaspoons of dried, crushed leaves per cup of boiling water. Steep ten minutes. Drink up to two cups a day. When using commercial products, follow the package directions.

If you live in the South or on the West Coast and have access to eucalyptus leaves, place a handful in boiling water and inhale the steamy vapor. For an herbal bath, wrap a handful of leaves in a cloth and run bathwater over it.

You can use a few drops of eucalyptus oil in boiling water or in the bath as an inhalant, but never ingest the oil. When the oil is taken internally, it is highly poisonous. Fatalities have been reported from ingestion of as little as a teaspoonful.

Eucalyptus oil is considered nonirritating to the skin, but sensitive individuals may develop a rash. If your skin gets red or irritated from the oil, discontinue its use.

Fennel

Comfort for New Parents

You're at an Indian restaurant waiting to be seated when you notice a small bowl of fennel seeds on a table by the door. You wonder what they're for, and before you know it, you're entertaining yourself with possibilities: An air freshener? Seasoning for the mango chutney? Something to be tossed over your shoulder for good luck?

The answer: The seeds are meant to be chewed in order to relieve gas, says Ara H. DerMarderosian, Ph.D., professor of pharmacognosy and medicinal chemistry at Philadelphia College of Pharmacy and Science. Through the ages, as far back as the ancient Romans, fennel has had a reputation as a flatulence reliever.

Historically, fennel has also been used to strengthen eyesight, relieve stomach upset, stimulate milk production in nursing mothers and promote menstruation. And those were just a few of its uses. It was reputed to be so effective, in fact, that an old Welsh

Potential Healing Power
May help: • **Alleviate gas** • **Relieve colic**

doctor once proclaimed that "He who sees fennel and gathers it not, is not a man, but a devil!"

Yet few of the historical uses of fennel have been scientifically substantiated. Its reputation as an aid for expelling gas is probably the most sound claim to date.

Possible Cure for Colic

A 1993 study conducted in Israel provides some support for the traditional use of fennel to relieve colic in infants. Researchers gave an herbal tea preparation containing fennel to 33 colicky babies and a nontherapeutic (placebo) drink to 35 other colicky infants for seven days. The researchers concluded that colic was eliminated in more of the babies who received herbal tea than in those who received the placebo drink.

Although the study is far from conclusive, it can't hurt to try giving fennel tea to a colicky baby. "It's worth a try, because colic is such a complex thing," says Dr. DerMarderosian.

To make fennel tea, steep ⅓ teaspoon of crushed fennel seed in a cup of boiling water.

Make sure you let the tea cool sufficiently before giving it to an infant. And, of course, if you're feeling a little gassy, you might want to try the tea yourself. Or you can do as the Indians do and nibble on a handful of fennel seeds—they have a pleasant, licorice-like flavor.

Fenugreek

Help for High Cholesterol

From ancient times through the late nineteenth century, fenugreek played a major role in herbal healing. Then it fell by the wayside. Now things are once again looking up for the herb whose taste is an odd combination of bitter celery and maple syrup. Modern scientific research has found that fenugreek can help reduce cholesterol levels, control diabetes and minimize the symptoms of menopause.

The ancient Greeks fed this herb to horses and cattle. The Romans then started using it, too, calling it "Greek hay." (In Latin, "Greek hay" is *foenum-graecum*, and that evolved into "fenugreek.") As fenugreek spread around the ancient Mediterranean, physicians learned that its seeds, like many seeds, contain a gummy substance called mucilage. Mixed with water, mucilage expands and becomes a gelatinous soother for irritated tissues.

In India, the herb was incorporated into curry blends. India's traditional Ayurvedic physicians prescribed it to nursing mothers to increase their milk. In American folk medicine, fenugreek was considered a potent menstruation promoter. It became a key ingredient in Lydia E. Pinkham's Vegetable Compound— one of nineteenth-century America's most popular patent medicines for "female weakness" (menstrual discomforts). Today, fenugreek is most widely used in

Potential Healing Power
May help: • Minimize symptoms of menopause • Relieve constipation • Control diabetes • Reduce cholesterol • Soothe sore throat pain and coughs • Ease minor indigestion • Relieve diarrhea

the United States as a source of imitation maple flavor. But this may change as its medicinal value becomes better known.

Almost a century after Lydia Pinkham's death, scientists have confirmed that fenugreek seeds contain chemicals (diosgenin and estrogenic isoflavones) similar to the female sex hormone estrogen. Loss of estrogen causes menopausal symptoms, so adding fenugreek to the diet might help minimize them. Estrogen can also cause breast swelling. "One woman told me her breasts grew larger after she started eating fenugreek sprouts," says James A. Duke, Ph.D., a botanist retired from the U.S. Department of Agriculture and author of *The CRC Handbook of Medicinal Herbs.*

Cholesterol Buster . . . and More

Several studies have shown that fenugreek reduces cholesterol in laboratory animals, and Indian researchers have shown the same effect in people with high cholesterol levels. The people in one Indian study added about four ounces a day of powdered fenugreek seeds to their diet for 20 days. During that time their total cholesterol levels and their levels of low-density lipoprotein (LDL, or "bad") cholesterol fell significantly. At the same time their high-density lipoprotein (HDL, or "good") cholesterol levels remained unaffected. "There's no question that fenugreek reduces cholesterol," says Daniel B. Mowrey, Ph.D., director of the American Phytotherapy Research Laboratory in Salt Lake City, Utah, and author of *The Scientific Validation of Herbal Medicine.*

Fenugreek also "has great promise in alleviating Type II (non-insulin-dependent) diabetes," says Dr. Duke. And according to one study, it may also help people with Type I (insulin-dependent) diabetes. For ten days, Indian researchers added about four ounces of powdered fenugreek seeds a day to the diets of people with Type I diabetes, which requires daily insulin injections. The injections, however, did not entirely eliminate a key sign of the illness, sugar in their urine. With fenugreek added to their diet, their urinary sugar levels fell by 54 percent.

Fenugreek's soothing mucilage can also help relieve sore throat pain, cough and minor indigestion. "Because its mucilage expands in the gut, it also adds bulk to the stool," says Bernie Olin, Pharm.D., editor of *The Lawrence Review of Natural Products*, a St. Louis–based newsletter that summarizes scientific research on the medicinal value of herbs. "As a result, it can help treat constipation and diarrhea."

To make a medicinal tea, gently boil two teaspoons of mashed seeds per cup of water, then simmer for ten minutes. Drink up to three cups a day. To improve the flavor, you can add sugar, honey, lemon, anise or peppermint.

Fenugreek is considered safe. But several of the conditions it helps—diabetes, elevated cholesterol and menopausal symptoms—require professional care. If you'd like to use this herb in addition to standard therapies, consult your physician.

Feverfew

Powerful Migraine Mauler

Despite its name, feverfew won't get rid of a fever. In fact, if today's scientists could rename this plant, they might want to dub it migraine-few.

In the 1980s, several studies done in the United Kingdom showed that people who regularly suffer from migraine headaches often find relief with feverfew. In the studies, migraine sufferers who chewed fresh feverfew leaves or took capsules of dried, ground leaves experienced fewer and less severe headaches.

The key to this effect, researchers believe, is parthenolide, a compound in feverfew that helps control the expansion and contraction of blood vessels in the brain. The unpleasant symptoms of migraine— nausea, throbbing head pain and sensitivity to light— apparently occur when blood vessels in the brain overreact, contracting and expanding abnormally.

This doesn't mean, though, that you can reach for feverfew to relieve a migraine.

"Feverfew has no beneficial effect on migraine attacks once they're in gear," says Varro E. Tyler, Ph.D., professor of pharmacognosy at Purdue University School of Pharmacy in West Lafayette, Indiana, and author of *The Honest Herbal.* "It works as a preventive, and that means taking it regularly over a long period."

Researchers suspect that feverfew may also help combat menstrual cramps and arthritic inflammation, although these uses are not as well substantiated.

Using Feverfew

Prescription medications are available for migraines, but they don't work for everybody. According to Daniel B. Mowrey, Ph.D., director of the American Phytotherapy Research Laboratory in Salt Lake City, Utah, and author of *The Scientific Validation of Herbal Medicine,* "The people feverfew works best for are usually those who don't respond to any other form of medication."

To duplicate the doses used in the migraine research, says Dr. Mowrey, "most people must eat a leaf or two or take a capsule or two each day." That's assuming you're getting perfectly potent feverfew, and that could prove difficult.

"The problem with feverfew in the United

Potential Healing Power

May help:
- Prevent migraine headaches
- Relieve arthritis
- Ease menstrual cramps

States," says Dr. Tyler, "is that you're very unlikely to get a quality product." Several investigators, he points out, have tested commercial feverfew preparations, such as tablets or extracts, and found that they contain little or no active ingredient.

For this reason, Dr. Tyler suggests taking more than the recommended dosage of any store-bought feverfew preparation to increase the odds of getting an adequate dose of the active ingredient, parthenolide. He recommends taking up to six 300- to 400-milligram tablets of the herb daily. Taking this much feverfew in tablet form is perfectly safe, he says.

You can also grow your own supply of fresh feverfew, says Dr. Mowrey. In fact, he suspects that whole feverfew leaves may work better than taking the active ingredient in concentrated form. "The research suggests strongly that the whole leaf has to be used," he says. "In some studies, people who just chewed on the leaf had better results than those who used pills filled with ground, dried plant material or an extract."

There is one potential drawback to eating feverfew leaves: They may cause irritation or ulcers of the lips, tongue and lining of the mouth. Otherwise, feverfew is generally considered safe. (If chewing feverfew leaves irritates your mouth, discontinue use immediately.)

It's also a good idea to steer clear of feverfew altogether if you are allergic to chamomile, chrysanthemum and other members of the daisy family. And since feverfew may also affect the clotting components of blood, people with a clotting disorder or those who take anti-clotting drugs probably shouldn't take it. And, just to be on the safe side, pregnant women should also avoid it.

Ginger

Spicy Weapon against Nausea

A beloved spice in kitchens around the world, ginger can do more than perk up food and beverages. It has proven merit for fighting nausea and may hold promise for the treatment of other conditions as well.

Ginger looks like a root, but botanically it is a rhizome, or underground stem. Cooks use it as a seasoning in various forms—sliced fresh, candied or powdered. But when it's used as a medicine, its pungency limits how much can be taken in one dose. Thanks to the invention of the gelatin capsule, more potent and convenient formulations of powdered ginger can now be used medicinally.

Spin Control

It's rare for an herbal remedy to be taken seriously in the pages of a major medical journal, but in 1982 ginger got the nod as an effective preventive for motion sickness from the prestigious British medical journal *Lancet.*

Daniel B. Mowrey, Ph.D., director of the American Phytotherapy Research Laboratory in Salt Lake City, Utah, and author of *The Scientific Validation of Herbal Medicine*, and a colleague compared the effects of pow-

Potential Healing Power

May help:
- Prevent motion sickness
- Fight nausea and diarrhea from stomach flu
- Relieve gas and indigestion

dered ginger to a standard dose of the over-the-counter antihistamine dimenhydrinate (Dramamine) in 36 college students who had a strong tendency to get motion sickness. After being spun in a tilted rotating chair, the ginger-treated students experienced less nausea and vertigo than the Dramamine-treated group. As a bonus, ginger causes none of the sleepy side effects associated with Dramamine and other antihistamines.

Nausea is a complex reaction involving various areas of the brain as well as the digestive tract, says Dr. Mowrey. Ginger appears to work directly on the stomach as well as on the brain to calm the heaves, he says.

In addition to its usefulness in battling motion sickness, ginger can also help reduce the nausea and diarrhea that often accompany stomach flu, says Dr. Mowrey.

All of these research findings bear out traditional uses of ginger in Chinese medicine to relieve indigestion and gas.

A Warming Trend

Other uses for ginger, although less firmly proven, have been suggested by various researchers. Scattered reports have linked ginger with relief of headaches, lowering of high blood cholesterol, reduction of rheumatoid arthritis symptoms and prevention of stomach ulcers.

A significant—and therapeutic—amount of ginger may be ingested by eating ginger-spiced food or drinking ginger ale (at least the kind flavored with real ginger, not a synthetic flavoring). Ditto for a cup of ginger tea made with a teaspoon of grated fresh root or dried powder. But to take ginger for motion sickness as needed at sea or on the road, capsules containing powdered ginger are quicker and easier.

In Dr. Mowrey's experiment, the dose (taken before motion began) was 940 milligrams, or about two standard ginger capsules. But he has a simpler guideline for knowing how much ginger to take to obtain results: "If you don't taste a little ginger on your breath or in your throat about five minutes after swallowing the capsule, you haven't taken enough."

There have been several scientific reports that ginger can help relieve morning sickness, including cases so severe that the women required hospital care. So far, there is no evidence that ginger has any adverse effects on an unborn child, but the risk has never been subjected to rigorous study. Herbal authorities say that a few ginger pills in the morning to quell nausea are probably safe, but just a few may not be effective—and higher doses increase the small but unknown risk. Play it safe. If you're pregnant, don't take any medicine or supplement—including ginger—without the consent of your obstetrician.

Ginkgo

Asian Guard against Aging

Talk about late bloomers! Ginkgo, the oldest living tree species on earth, has been used medicinally by the Chinese for some 4,000 years. Yet only in the last two decades have Western medical researchers found evidence that ginkgo may offer hope for a host of age-related problems.

Ginkgo trees, also known as maidenhair trees, are often planted on city streets. The tree's fruit smells awful when decomposed and can cause skin irritation, but the almondlike seed within is prized as a commodity in Asian markets.

It is the ginkgo's pretty, fan-shaped leaf, not its foul fruit, that excites scientists these days. Although little known in this country outside of health food stores, a concentrated extract of the plant has been the number-one prescription drug in Germany, where it is used to help asthma and circulation problems. And unlike many plant-based therapeutic agents, "ginkgo preparations have been extensively tested in people, not just in animals and test tubes," says Norman R. Farnsworth, Ph.D., director of the Program for Collaborative Research in the Pharmaceutical Sciences at the University of Illinois at Chicago.

Powerful Medicine

What's in ginkgo extract, and what can it do? The active constituents include unique compounds called ginkgolides. One of these compounds, ginkgolide B, has been shown to suppress a clot-promoting substance in the human body called platelet activating factor, or PAF. Since PAF is a key player in body processes such as allergic inflammation and asthma, the disease-fighting potential of ginkgo is intriguing.

This and other substances in ginkgo extract have shown various benefits for the ills of old age, especially those resulting from decreased blood supply to the brain and other parts of the body. These effects are believed to stem from ginkgo's ability to dilate arteries and capillaries, the tiny blood vessels that nourish the body's tissues.

Perhaps most exciting is ginkgo's potential for improving short-term memory loss and depression in elderly people. "The research on ginkgo and Alzheimer's disease is producing extremely good re-

Potential Healing Power

May help:
- Improve tinnitus (ringing in the ears)
- Relieve symptoms of Alzheimer's disease, including short-term memory loss and depression
- Reduce inflammation due to asthma and allergies
- Fight damage from stroke
- Ease outbreaks of multiple sclerosis
- Lessen symptoms of peripheral vascular disease and Raynaud's disease

sults in France and Germany," says Daniel B. Mowrey, Ph.D., director of the American Phytotherapy Research Laboratory in Salt Lake City, Utah, and author of *The Scientific Validation of Herbal Medicine*. "It seems that the earlier you catch the disease, the greater the chances that you can reverse it by taking ginkgo extract."

The extract has also reduced symptoms of peripheral vascular disease and Raynaud's disease, two painful conditions involving impaired circulation in the feet and hands. And "there are many clinical studies showing it can reduce tinnitus, or ringing in the ears, which affects many older people," according to Dr. Farnsworth.

German research performed on laboratory rats confirmed previous evidence that ginkgolide B may minimize the devastation of stroke. And a French study on humans showed that it may even allay bouts of multiple sclerosis.

Rx: Going Ginkgo

Remember, though, the only well-demonstrated benefits of ginkgo have been from a concentrated extract, not from the leaves themselves. Such extracts are available in the United States, and they are labeled as food supplements, not drugs, in accordance with U.S. regulations. Regular use of such products is widespread in Europe, according to Varro E. Tyler, Ph.D., professor of pharmacognosy at Purdue University School of Pharmacy in West Lafayette, Indiana, and author of *The Honest Herbal*.

Ginkgo extract is generally considered safe, says Dr. Tyler, although it has been noted to cause some generally mild side effects, including restlessness and digestive upset. If you experience such symptoms, he advises, discontinue use. And since ginkgo also affects the body's clotting mechanism, Dr. Tyler warns, use it cautiously if you take anti-clotting medications, including aspirin, or have a clotting disorder.

Dr. Tyler also warns against ginkgo hype aimed at older folks. "While ginkgo has apparently been effective in treating ailments associated with decreased cerebral blood flow in old age," he says, "claims that ginkgo extract will 'reverse the aging process' and increase longevity are, of course, unproven."

Ginseng

The Inscrutable Root

In 1711, a Jesuit missionary stationed in China gave the West its first glimpse of ginseng. "Nobody can imagine that the Chinese and Tartars would set so high a value on this root, if it did not constantly produce a good effect," he wrote. Surely it was only a matter of time, he said, before European pharmacists figured out how to use this age-old remedy.

Almost 300 years later, ginseng, perhaps the most researched herb on earth, remains a mystery. Some claim it's a panacea, others insist it's worthless—and

Potential Healing Power
May help:
• **Relieve stress**
• **Improve stamina**
• **Regulate blood pressure**
• **Enhance immunity**

medical researchers suggest that the power of ginseng, if any, may lie in its complexity.

Name That Herb

Ginseng refers to at least three different plants. The mother of all ginseng is the Asian variety, *Panax ginseng*, prescribed in 2,000-year-old Chinese texts to "quiet the spirit and increase wisdom." A close cousin is American ginseng (*P. quinquefolius*). Just to confuse matters, a distantly related plant called Eleuthero, or Siberian ginseng, has recently become popular as a cheap substitute for "real" ginseng.

All three types of ginseng are traditionally used as tonics—to strengthen and regulate body functions and thus treat a host of ailments. Some of the fleshy roots look vaguely like a human figure, which possibly explains their reputation as a body-wide cure-all.

Is there anything to this tradition? Many scientists have tried to test the powers of ginseng, with results as frustrating as a Chinese puzzle. "I'm sure ginseng does *something*, but there's so much conflicting information that it's impossible to say just what this herb does in human beings," says Norman R. Farnsworth, Ph.D., director of the Program for Collaborative Research in the Pharmaceutical Sciences at the University of Illinois at Chicago.

Experts agree that ginseng contains a variety of compounds called ginsenosides. And various ginsenosides have been shown in test-tube and animal studies to have contradictory effects. Some of these chemicals appear to raise blood pressure; others seem to lower it. Some act as sedatives, others as stimulants.

Some herbalists argue that the complex nature of ginseng is exactly what makes it a good tonic—that is, a remedy that helps the body achieve balance, warding off damage from disease and other stresses. A more scientific term for a tonic is *adaptogen*—something that helps the body adapt (for example, by regulating temperature or blood pressure up or down toward normal).

Studies have shown that substances found in Asian and American ginseng may indeed bolster the immune system and have a positive effect on conditions ranging from diabetes to high blood pressure.

As for Siberian ginseng, it is widely used by Russians, including cosmonauts and athletes, to improve stamina and resist stress. And Russian research offers evidence that some of these effects may be real.

Despite all the research that's been done on ginseng, it will still take some large, well-done studies on humans to confirm its benefits, says Dr. Farnsworth.

Using the Mystery Herb

Many American products are simply labeled "ginseng," but Chinese medicine differentiates among the three types. For example, Asian ginseng has "warming" properties, and should be used "to reinvigorate the body, as after a long illness," says Albert Leung, Ph.D., a pharmacognosist and author of *Chinese Healing Foods and Herbs*. But American ginseng is "cooling," he says, and should be used by people who are "overheated and excited."

Unfortunately, debating such fine points may sometimes be moot—because there's no guarantee that a ginseng product contains any ginseng at all! Since ginseng is so costly, packagers are tempted to dilute or substitute cheaper ingredients. One 1978 study analyzed 54 ginseng products and found that 25 percent contained no ginseng whatsoever. Your best bet is to buy ginseng products only from a reputable source.

Ginseng consumption seems to have few reported side effects. As with any herb, however, possible risk increases with higher intake over longer periods. If you decide to take any ginseng product, start low and go slow.

Dried ginseng root may be powdered and taken in capsule form or brewed as a tea. Extracts are also available in various formulations for use internally and externally, and these should include instructions for proper dosage. As with any herb, experts advise against taking ginseng if you are pregnant or nursing, unless you're under the care of a medical specialist.

Goldenseal

Yellow Cure for Sore Throats

Cherokee warriors once ground goldenseal's roots as a source of bright yellow face paint. And Cherokee medicine men used the herb medicinally, applying it to arrow wounds and inflamed eyes. Early American colonists also learned to appreciate goldenseal—as a digestive tonic, as an astringent rinse for sore throats and canker sores and to stop bleeding after childbirth.

A wildflower of North American forests, goldenseal soon leaped the Atlantic and became popular in Europe as well. To this day, it remains a favorite among herbalists throughout the Western world, who still use it to treat eye irritations, minor skin wounds and indigestion. They also swear by goldenseal as an infection fighter and immune system booster.

But does science bear out folklore as to the herb's medicinal powers?

The effects of goldenseal on human beings have not been extensively studied. But chemical analysis has turned up two main active chemicals in the roots. These alkaloid compounds—berberine and hydrastine—have a wide array of effects on the human body.

Berberine reduces hemorrhaging and is a powerful antiseptic, medical experts say. In the gastrointestinal tract, it has been shown to fight diarrhea-causing mi-

Potential Healing Power

May help:
- Soothe sore throat
- Relieve indigestion
- Kill germs internally and externally
- Ease red, tired eyes
- Prevent and treat diarrhea caused by microorganisms

croorganisms, including *Giardia*—a parasite common in water supplies around the world—and even cholera. Berberine also acts as a mild local anesthetic on mucous membranes. This lends scientific confirmation to the use of goldenseal tea as a gargle to treat sore throat.

Hydrastine has long been used as an ingredient in commercial eyewashes. This compound constricts tiny blood vessels—an action that may "get the red out" of tired eyes but may also cause a rise in blood pressure throughout the body when the compound is taken internally.

Unproven Remedy with a Potent Reputation

Overall, this herb's safety and effectiveness for various health problems remain unclear—at least until further study is done. Although goldenseal would make any herbalist's list of "greatest hits," there is still controversy and disagreement as to what it's good for and in what forms and dosages.

"Goldenseal tea may be a modestly effective astringent for sore mouth and lips," says Varro E. Tyler,

Ph.D., professor of pharmacognosy at Purdue University School of Pharmacy in West Lafayette, Indiana, and author of *The Honest Herbal*. But as for taking it internally, he warns: "Unless you take doses large enough to be nearly toxic, the effects are too uncertain to be useful."

Although there is little evidence of harm caused by taking goldenseal, if you're going to use goldenseal internally, it's a good idea to take it under the supervision of a doctor who knows about herbs. And don't take goldenseal, or an herbal blend containing it, if you are pregnant or have high blood pressure. (In addition to its potential for raising blood pressure, the herb contains compounds that can stimulate contractions of the uterus.)

To make a tea that you can use for sore throats, pour a cup of boiling water over one teaspoon of the dried herb. Allow the tea to cool until lukewarm and use it as a gargle.

Gotu Kola

Far Eastern Wound Healer

This creeping, marsh-loving plant isn't well known outside its native range of China, India and the South Pacific. In those regions, however, gotu kola has quite a reputation. In China, it's considered the

Potential Healing Power

May help:
- **Heal wounds**
- **Improve circulation in the legs**
- **Relieve anxiety**
- **Promote sleep**

herb of choice to promote longevity, in part because it was used regularly by the Chinese herbalist Li Ching Yun, who, legend says, lived to celebrate his 256th birthday.

In India, gotu kola is known as the herb of enlightenment. "This plant is called *brambi*, or 'greatest of the great,'" says Jay L. Glaser, M.D., medical director of the Maharishi Ayurvedic Health Center in Lancaster, Massachusetts. (Ayurvedic medicine is the traditional medicine of India.) "Gotu kola's most important use is to bring the nervous system to such an extreme degree of refinement that the individual can see his or her nature as unbounded and infinite—in other words, to become enlightened," says Dr. Glaser.

Gotu kola is also used in Ayurvedic medicine as a cure for agitation, memory loss, anxiety, insomnia, epilepsy and hyperactivity, Dr. Glaser says.

As intriguing as these claims and uses may sound, gotu kola has yet to be checked out in any organized way or with modern scientific techniques. But the two most common forms of the herb, *Centella asiatica* and *Hydrocotyle asiatica*, are known to contain several active ingredients that apparently do offer anti-inflammatory, antibacterial and sedative effects. "This herb has been described as representing an entire apothecary shop, and indeed it has many, many uses," says Daniel B. Mowrey, Ph.D., director of the American Phytotherapy Research Laboratory in Salt Lake City, Utah, and author of *The Scientific Validation of Herbal Medicine*.

In India, Indonesia and Europe, gotu kola has traditionally been used (and is still employed) to promote healing of tissue, including surgical wounds, burns, tears that occur during childbirth, anal fissures and skin ulcers, Dr. Mowrey says. "Clinical studies done overseas indicate that standardized extracts of gotu kola can greatly aid wound repair," he says. And, he says, it works equally well when taken orally or put on the skin. The herb apparently enhances cells' ability to manufacture protein and thus stimulates the growth of new tissue, he says.

Gotu kola also seems to help improve blood flow through the veins in the legs. In one study, it improved such symptoms as heaviness in the lower legs, numbness, nighttime cramps, swelling and distended veins. "It's thought to help keep veins strong and resistant to bulging by promoting the growth of connective tissues, which helps keep vein walls strong," Dr. Mowrey says.

Gotu kola contains compounds that researchers are very interested in right now—flavonoids, or terpenes. Some of this group of biochemicals are known to have anti-cancer activity. "Whether gotu kola contains those particular flavonoids that offer protection from cancer remains to be seen," Dr. Mowrey says.

Exotic but Available

You can find gotu kola at many health food stores. Capsules containing powdered *H. asiatica*, the weaker variety of gotu kola, are most commonly available. "People using this herb for health maintenance usually take two to four 400-milligram capsules a day of *H. asiatica*, which is the cheaper variety," Dr. Mowrey explains. The stronger kind, *C. asiatica*, is available as capsules or extract. "The extract is more expensive and is usually reserved for treating serious illness such as epilepsy," Dr. Mowrey says. People using the extract for a medical condition generally take one to two ounces a day, Dr. Glaser says.

The Food and Drug Administration considers gotu kola an herb of "undefined safety." Two side effects are possible—sedation and skin rash. If you are thinking about taking gotu kola for a medical condition, it's best to talk with a health professional who's familiar with herbs to determine whether it is a wise choice for you, Dr. Glaser says.

Guarana

A Potent Source of Energy

With a healthy population of poisonous spiders, plants and snakes as neighbors, the folks who live in the Amazon Basin need all the help they can get to stay alert and on their toes. And they get a major assist from guarana, a woody vine native to that region of the world.

"A cup of the beverage made from guarana has three times more caffeine than a cup of coffee," says William J. Keller, Ph.D., professor and head of the Division of Medicinal Chemistry and Pharmaceutics at the Northeast Louisiana University School of Pharmacy in Monroe. "People in South America either chew a spoonful of the seeds or crush the seeds with a mortar and pestle, add a sprinkle of water and mix up a paste. The dried paste is then used to make a hot beverage like coffee.

"Back in the 1970s, the dried paste was made into tablet form and sold under the name 'Zoom!'" he adds. "One tablet had the caffeine equivalent of four or five tablets of Nō-Dōz."

Other than keeping you moving in a dangerous environment, guarana may also have the ability to keep your red blood cells moving when they have a tendency to clump together and trigger a heart attack.

In a laboratory study conducted at the University of Sao Paulo in Brazil, researchers found that guarana extract reduces the clumping of red blood cells in rabbits anywhere from 27 to 37 percent.

Does it do the same in humans? Nobody knows for sure, the researchers report. They're still trying to figure out exactly what it is that keeps the blood cells from clumping together. While guarana may hold po-

---

Potential Healing Power

May help:
• Prevent drowsiness
• Reduce risk of heart attack

tential as a heart protector, it's still too soon to recommend it.

What about using guarana to stay awake? While you can still purchase the herb at health food stores, you might want to reach for a cup of coffee instead. Guarana packs a mighty potent dose of caffeine—enough to give many people the jitters.

Hawthorn

Hope for Heart Health

The hawthorn, a small thorny tree belonging to the rose family, has long been a symbol of hope—ancient Greek brides carried it on their wedding day. Herbalists have kept it in their repertoire for thousands of years, but only since the turn of this century has it been explored for a truly hopeful purpose: to heal the human heart.

The small reddish fruits of the hawthorn are used as food in many countries. In the nineteenth century, an Irish doctor included them in a "secret remedy" for heart disease. His discovery was popularized in the 1890s by a group of American physicians known as the Eclectics. These doctors used hawthorn preparations to treat cardiac troubles such as weak heartbeat and angina. It seems they may have been onto something.

Over the past 80 years, research on both animals and people has confirmed that hawthorn has positive effects on the cardiovascular (heart and blood vessel) system, probably through the action of plant pigments called flavonoids.

Hawthorn seems to work in two main ways, according to Varro E. Tyler, Ph.D., professor of pharmacognosy at Purdue University School of Pharmacy in West Lafayette, Indiana, and author of *The Honest Herbal*. "First, it dilates the blood vessels, especially the coronary arteries that nourish the heart muscle. This may help lower blood pressure and reduce angina," he explains. When the arteries dilate, or open wider, pressure throughout the blood vessel system is lowered—just like opening the nozzle wider on a garden hose. "Second," says Dr. Tyler, "hawthorn seems to have a direct positive action on the heart itself when taken over the long term. Apparently, it's a mild and harmless heart tonic."

So why aren't more people using hawthorn? In Germany they are. German pharmacies carry three dozen hawthorn preparations, both prescription and nonprescription, to treat heart-related ailments, says Dr. Tyler. There, hawthorn is recommended to treat very mild cases of circulatory disorders or in addition to therapy with stronger heart drugs such as digitalis.

Potential Healing Power

May help:
- Regulate blood pressure
- Reduce angina pain

Don't Doctor Your Own Heart

Given these observations—plus the fact that hawthorn has no record of dangerous side effects—why shouldn't the millions of Americans with heart and blood vessel problems take hawthorn pills and extracts, which are available in health food stores?

Because with cardiovascular problems, there's no good reason for self-doctoring, say herbal experts. "People who dose themselves usually do so because they've diagnosed themselves—and with a vital system like the heart and blood vessels, that can be a very dangerous thing to do," warns Dr. Tyler. "For this reason, I don't recommend self-treatment with hawthorn."

"Don't fiddle around with the heart," warns Norman Farnsworth, Ph.D., director of the Program for Collaborative Research in the Pharmaceutical Sciences at the University of Illinois at Chicago and a heart attack survivor. "There are well-established synthetic drugs available for cardiac trouble, and some herbal products could possibly interact with them. Taking them along with prescription medications wouldn't be wise—I wouldn't do it myself."

If you're already under a doctor's care for heart or blood vessel problems, you might ask about adding a hawthorn preparation to other forms of therapy—but don't be surprised if your doctor is unfamiliar with the herb. Most American doctors don't know hawthorn.

And if you take any prescription heart medications or blood pressure drugs, play it safe and avoid adding any herbal remedies to the mix, advises Dr. Farnsworth.

Horehound

A Traditional Cough Remedy

O nce upon a time, Europeans believed horehound would help ward off witches' spells. But whatever the herb's anti-ghoul properties, they apparently weren't powerful enough to prevent the Food and Drug Administration (FDA) from casting a spell over horehound in 1989. Over the protests of herbalists that year, the FDA ruled horehound ineffective against coughs and banned it from over-the-counter cough remedies.

That was news to traditional herbalists. They've been recommending horehound to treat coughs for literally thousands of years. You might think the FDA ruling was the end of the story, but it's not. You can still buy the herb, you can still buy horehound candies, and some herbal experts say the final word has not yet been said on this topic.

David P. Carew, Ph.D., professor emeritus of medicinal and natural products chemistry at the University of Iowa in Iowa City, for example, actually whips up his own tasty, old-fashioned horehound candy at home. "I like the flavor of horehound myself," says Dr. Carew. "I also think there's some mucus-ejecting action in horehound, but I'm sure it

Potential Healing Power

May help:
• Relieve coughs

all depends on how strong the extract is that you put in."

Horehound's phlegm-evicting component is thought to be released when the herb is cooked. Called marrubiin, this chemical apparently irritates the lining of the throat, causing horehound's expectorant action, according to Varro E. Tyler, Ph.D., professor of pharmacognosy at Purdue University School of Pharmacy in West Lafayette, Indiana, and author of *The Honest Herbal*.

During one study, marrubiin was found to increase the production of bile in laboratory animals, says John Michael Edwards, Ph.D., associate dean of the School of Pharmacy at the University of Connecticut at Storrs. "Presumably this means it would stimulate all sorts of secretions," says Dr. Edwards. "Think of it this way: Something that increases one secretion is likely to stimulate others."

Horehound has never been just a cough remedy. It has had other uses over the years as well, from luring bees to gardens and adding a flavorful punch to English ales to featured status as a bitter herb during Jewish Passover. One group of physicians in nineteenth-century America also prescribed it for colds, asthma, intestinal worms and menstrual complaints. None of these uses has been scientifically investigated, however.

Old-Fashioned Relief?

If you'd like to try horehound tea, pour a cup of boiling water over one teaspoon of dried horehound leaves and steep for ten minutes. Sweeten to taste. The candies are hard to find, and if you do find them, you'll see that they no longer come with a medicinal label.

You can judge for yourself whether the ancients were right about horehound's ability to relieve a cough. You can also enjoy the candies just as a treat, although the sweet/bitter taste is unusual, to say the least.

Hyssop

Potential Anti-AIDS Weapon

Hyssop has a history of medicinal use as old as the Bible. But at least one study shows the herb could serve as a potent weapon in the very modern fight against AIDS.

The investigation into hyssop's anti-AIDS properties began after a 29-year-old female heroin addict suffering from the virus arrived for treatment at North Shore University Hospital in Manhassett, New York. Among other ailments at the time, the woman had

Potential Healing Power
May help: • Treat AIDS-related conditions   • Relieve congestion due to colds   • Soothe respiratory problems   • Loosen phlegm

contracted Kaposi's sarcoma—a deadly cancer characterized by bluish-red lesions that frequently develops in people who have AIDS.

A year later, a checkup revealed that the woman's skin lesions had improved "significantly" and she was feeling "much better," says Willi Kreis, M.D., Ph.D., an oncologist at North Shore University Hospital and research professor at Cornell Medical College in New York City.

The source of her improvement was a mystery—until the woman's mother told researchers her daughter had been drinking an old Jamaican tea remedy made from hyssop and a few other herbs. What were the doctors to think? They weren't used to seeing Kaposi's sarcoma get better. In fact, until the time of her death from AIDS-related pneumonia, the woman continued to drink her tea, and her Kaposi's sarcoma continued to regress, says Dr. Kreis. "After we heard that, we decided we had to study hyssop," he says.

The team's lab work, chronicled in a leading medical journal, seems to confirm hyssop's preliminary promise, says Dr. Kreis. "Our study was done just with tissue cultures in the laboratory, but hyssop was very effective as an antiviral, anti-HIV treatment in the test systems that we used," he says. (Doctors say that the human immunodeficiency virus—HIV—causes AIDS.)

It Fights Colds, Too

Of course, ancient herbalists weren't using hyssop against AIDS, but they were enthusiastic about its healing properties. A member of the mint family, hyssop has had advocates since antiquity. Among them were two of the biggest names in ancient medicine, Hippocrates and Galen. Both suggested hyssop for bronchitis. Other folk uses of hyssop include treating coughs, colds, hoarseness, fevers, sore throats and herpes.

An ingredient in some liqueurs, hyssop's leaves and flowers contain a volatile oil that gives it a bitter taste and strong odor, says William J. Keller, Ph.D., professor and head of the Division of Medicinal Chemistry and Pharmaceutics at Northeast Louisiana University School of Pharmacy in Monroe. "That's one thing generally common to mint plants: They produce a lot of volatile oil, the thing that gives spearmint and peppermint their characteristic flavor," he says. "As it turns out, a chemical in the volatile oil is good for treating irritations of the respiratory tract and congestion due to colds. It also acts as an expectorant."

To make hyssop tea, steep two teaspoons of the fresh or dried herb in a cup of boiling water. Add sugar, honey or lemon to taste.

Juniper

Nature's Ultimate Water Pill

If you occasionally enjoy a dry martini, you can thank juniper berries. Actually, you can thank a seventeenth-century Dutch physician named Franciscus de la Boe, otherwise known as Dr. Sylvius. Dr. Sylvius was well aware that juniper berries are a powerful diuretic that helps the body flush away excess water. And it was while trying to distill the essence of juniper berries into alcohol that he inadvertently created gin.

His herbal concoction proved extremely popular, especially with the English, who didn't give two hoots that it was *supposed* to be medicinal.

The use of the oil from juniper berries as medicine goes way back. Egyptian doctors used it as a laxative as early as 1550 B.C. Since then, in various times and places, the oil has been used to treat an incredible variety of human ailments, everything from cancer and arthritis to gas and warts. Also appearing on this unlikely list: swelling, bronchitis, tuberculosis, gallstones, colic, heart failure, intestinal diseases, gonorrhea, gout, hysteria and back pain.

Over time, herbalists finally focused on the kidneys as the favored organ for treatment with juniper. They recommended the herb for kidney disease, kidney stones and inflamed kidneys.

Little Berries with a Powerful Punch

It wasn't until the current century that doctors discovered that juniper actually irritates the kidneys, says William J. Keller, Ph.D., professor and head of the Division of Medicinal Chemistry and Pharmaceutics at Northeast Louisiana University School of Pharmacy in Monroe. While juniper is a potent diuretic, it's actually harmful to anyone with a kidney problem. What's more, as little as six drops of the oil can have a toxic effect whether or not you have kidney disease.

That's why you should never just pick a handful of berries and munch, says Dr. Keller. "The safest way to use juniper oil is to buy it in health food stores as an ingredient in over-the-counter 'water pills.' And as long as you're not pregnant, just follow the dosage instructions on the label.

"Under no circumstances should a pregnant woman use juniper in any form," adds Dr. Keller. It's known to cause miscarriage.

The best use of juniper? Probably as the flavoring agent in gin-and-tonic, chuckles Dr. Keller. These days, there's just enough juniper oil to give the drink its characteristic flavor and smell, but not enough to have a pharmacological effect.

Potential Healing Power

May help:
• Reduce water retention

Kola

It's a Real Herb

Colas account for more than half of the enormous U.S. soft drink market. Yet few Americans know that the tropical nut that flavors cola has several medicinal benefits.

West Africans have used kola since prehistoric times for its stimulant effect, and no wonder—kola contains caffeine. In one 12-ounce can of cola, you'll find about 40 milligrams. For comparison, a 6-ounce cup of brewed coffee contains about 100 milligrams of caffeine, and a cup of instant coffee contains about 60.

When slaves brought kola to the New World, its stimulant action was adopted medicinally as an antidepressant pick-me-up. Pharmacists stocked it, including John Pemberton of Atlanta, who aspired to developing a kola-based "nerve tonic." Legend has it that in 1886, Pemberton mixed some sugar with extracts of kola and coca (the source of cocaine) in a three-legged brass pot in his backyard. He added carbonated water to his sweet syrup and created a refreshing drink that his bookkeeper dubbed Coca-Cola. Today, Coca-Cola is one of the best-known brand names in the world. Its formula has always been a closely guarded secret, but regardless of whether Coke ever contained cocaine, you can be sure that today its kick comes entirely from caffeine.

Soda with a Gentle Kick

As with coffee, kola's caffeine content accounts for both its medicinal benefits and its potential problems. On the plus side, caffeine increases the pain-relieving action of aspirin. It is also a stimulant that may open (dilate) the bronchial passages and temporarily increase athletic stamina. On the minus side, large amounts of caffeine can cause insomnia, jitters, irritability and upset stomach and, some experts say, may increase risk of heart attack. It's also addictive. Once you are accustomed to caffeine, sudden elimination often causes a headache that can last for several days.

"In moderate amounts—no more than 250 milligrams a day—caffeine is reasonably safe," says Varro E. Tyler, Ph.D., professor of pharmacognosy at Purdue University School of Pharmacy in West Lafayette, Indiana, and author of *The Honest Herbal*. "Most healthy people can consume up to that much before they need to get too concerned."

Cola beverages, although they tend to be loaded with sugar, are the most convenient way to consume this herb. But for a medicinal tea, add one to two tea-

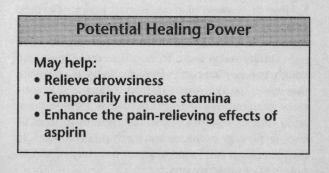

Potential Healing Power

May help:
- Relieve drowsiness
- Temporarily increase stamina
- Enhance the pain-relieving effects of aspirin

spoons of powdered kola nut to a cup of water. Bring to a boil and simmer ten minutes. Drink up to three cups a day.

Kola nut may be difficult to find in your neighborhood grocery store. Two suppliers that do stock it are Herb and Spice Collection, 3021 78th Street, P.O. Box 118, Norway, IA 52318-0118 and Nature's Herb Company, 1010 46th Street, Emeryville, CA 94608.

Licorice

Sweet-Tasting Ulcer Therapy

Say "licorice," and most people think of candy. But licorice is actually a potent and controversial herb. Just to confuse matters, not all licorice-flavored candy contains real licorice—some is artificially flavored.

Traditionally used to soothe sore throat and cough, real licorice comes from the roots of a tall plant that has been cultivated in both China and Europe since ancient times. Ancient herbalists, both Western and Chinese, used the sweet-tasting root to treat ulcers, respiratory problems and many other ailments. In fact, licorice is still found in about one-third of all Chinese herbal prescriptions.

Today, licorice is most widely used as flavoring in tobacco products. It may also be found in some throat lozenges, in European licorice candies and in some American candies.

Licorice owes its sweetness to glycyrrhizin, a compound 50 times sweeter than sugar. Every so often, a medical journal will report serious illness from an "overdose" of real licorice. The overdose isn't from taking the herb, however. Usually it's from eating literally pounds of the candy or from swallowing saliva from licorice-laced chewing tobacco. Overdose symptoms include high blood pressure, weakness and water retention. The substance responsible for the herb's sweetness is also the culprit in overdose symptoms. Medical experts report that glycyrrhizin mimics a naturally occurring hormone that affects the body's metabolism and water content.

Powerful Ingredients

What about the positive side of the herb? Few people, after all, consume licorice candy by the pound.

During World War II, a Dutch doctor observed that licorice extract helped heal peptic ulcers but also caused swelling of the face and limbs. This discovery led to the widespread use of a licorice-based com-

Potential Healing Power
May help: • Soothe sore throat • Relieve coughs • Heal peptic ulcers

pound—carbenoxolone—to treat ulcers. In the 1970s, the discovery of safer and more effective anti-ulcer drugs knocked carbenoxolone, with its potentially dangerous side effects, out of the running.

Licorice as an ulcer remedy has refused to stay in the dustbin of medical history, however. When researchers removed glycyrrhizin from licorice root and then tested it again, they found that the root *still* healed ulcers. Clearly, there was healing power in some other component of licorice.

Today, some herbal practitioners remain enthusiastic about the anti-ulcer powers of this "safe," or *deglycyrrhizinated*, licorice, called DGL. "This product is wonderful for healing peptic ulcers," says Alan R. Gaby, M.D., a Baltimore physician who practices nutritional and natural medicine and is president of the American Holistic Medical Association. "In some studies it has worked about as well as standard anti-ulcer therapies like Tagamet and Zantac, for a lower cost and with virtually no risk."

Use with Caution

Because licorice—the real stuff, with glycyrrhizin—can cause such serious side effects in high doses, consume only modest amounts of any product labeled "real licorice." Limit your enjoyment to a few pieces. And, to be on the safe side, avoid all licorice products if you have high blood pressure, heart disease or glaucoma.

Ulcer treatment is not something you should undertake on your own. If you have ulcer symptoms, you should see your doctor, says Dr. Gaby, "but DGL is worth a try." If you'd like to use DGL, discuss it with your doctor.

And if you'd like to give the herb's traditional ability to soothe a sore throat a try, simply sprinkle a pinch of the powdered herb into hot water or tea.

Marshmallow

A Gooey Throat Soother

Floating in a steaming cup of cocoa or skewered on a sharp stick, marshmallows may seem like little more than glorified cream puffs—and rubbery ones at that. It's hard to believe that the sugary confections have a medicinal history.

Actually, our modern marshmallows—the buoyant white candy that made S'Mores famous—no longer contain the herb for which they were named.

Marshmallow, the herb, comes from a tall plant with a long root that grows (no surprise) in marshes. Nineteeth-century doctors cooked juice from the marshmallow plant's roots with egg whites and sugar and whipped them into a foamy meringue that later hardened, creating a medicinal candy used to soothe children's sore throats. This medicine proved popular with adults as well as children, mostly as a candy. Eventually, advanced manufacturing processes and improved texturing agents eliminated the need for the gooey root juice altogether.

Potential Healing Power

May help:
- Soothe sore throat
- Relieve coughs

The Power Is in the Slide

Centuries before marshmallow was ever used to make candy, physicians were prescribing preparations made from marshmallow roots, flowers and leaves for coughs and sore throats. In fact, the scientific name for marshmallow is *Althaea officinalis*, from the Greek word *althaea*, meaning "to heal."

As it turns out, the leaves, light pink flowers and roots of the marshmallow plant all contain a thick, gooey substance called mucilage.

"The mucilage can soothe irritation in your throat and help you stop coughing," says Heinz Rosler, Ph.D., associate professor of medicinal chemistry at the University of Maryland School of Pharmacy in Baltimore. In fact, when pitted against two other remedies in an Eastern European study of cough suppressants, marshmallow outperformed both. Teas containing marshmallow are commonly sold in Germany for this purpose, says Dr. Rosler.

Although the herb is not as widely available here, you can sometimes purchase marshmallow teas at health food stores. You can also make a tea by boiling ½ to 1 teaspoon of crushed root per cup of water for 10 to 15 minutes.

Meadowsweet

Aspirin from the Fields

Imagine your doctor dispensing a bouquet of small, creamy white flowers instead of aspirin every time your arthritis acts up.

It's actually not that farfetched. If nineteenth-century scientists had failed to unlock the secret of salicylic acid, you might well be picking up flowers from your doctor for things like arthritis, headaches and the flu.

That's because the bud of the meadowsweet plant naturally contains salicin, one form of the key ingredient in an aspirin tablet, says William J. Keller, Ph.D., professor and head of the Division of Medicinal Chemistry and Pharmaceutics at Northeast Louisiana University School of Pharmacy in Monroe. "Once the salicin from meadowsweet is in the stomach, it breaks down to create salicylic acid, and basically that's what happens when you take an aspirin," he explains.

For that reason, centuries-old uses for meadowsweet—for headaches, arthritis and the flu—seem justifiable, says Dr. Keller. "It definitely has an analgesic effect, and it lowers body temperature, so it's even good for fever."

Herbalists also give meadowsweet high marks as a remedy for heartburn, gastritis, peptic ulcers and urinary tract infections. There is as yet no scientific research to support these traditional uses, but research

Potential Healing Power

May help:
• Banish headache pain
• Relieve the aches of flu
• Ease arthritis pain
• Reduce fever

continues. Over the past few years, for example, Russian medical researchers have begun studying meadowsweet's suspected ability to inhibit blood clotting.

Have a Spot of Comfort

You can test meadowsweet's painkilling powers for yourself in the form of a tea. Add one to two teaspoons of the dried herb to a cup of boiling water and let it steep for ten minutes before drinking.

There's one traditional use of the herb that requires no scientific study to confirm. During the Middle Ages, the plant's almond-scented flowers were often strewn to improve the smell of rooms. (Back when farm animals shared living space with people, and people didn't bathe regularly, room-freshening herbs were far more important than they are today.) Meadowsweet smells just as good as it ever did—and, if you're lucky enough to have some growing in your area, the fresh wildflowers can *still* make a room smell absolutely wonderful.

Milk Thistle

Protection for the Liver

The milk thistle, a tall, spiny plant native to the Mediterranean, got its name from its milky sap—and from a legend that the plant's white-veined leaves resulted from a sprinkling of mother's milk from the Virgin Mary. (The legend accounts for its other name, Mary thistle, and its botanical name, *Silybum marianum*.)

This tale gave rise to a folk belief that the plant was good for nursing mothers. There is no proof that milk thistle helps breast-feeding. But it has shown dramatic results in healing liver problems.

Milk thistle has been used to treat the liver for some 2,000 years. In the first century A.D., the Roman naturalist Pliny wrote that the seedlike fruits of the milk thistle were "excellent for carrying off bile." Later herbalists also esteemed the herb as a liver healer. In the past two decades, research, conducted mainly in Europe, has proven them right.

The active substance in milk thistle seeds is called silymarin—a complex of various compounds that, according to medical researchers, not only protects the liver from damage due to toxins or disease but can actually regenerate liver tissue that's already in trouble.

"Silymarin is a powerful antioxidant," says Alan R. Gaby, M.D., a Baltimore physician who practices nutritional and natural medicine and is president of the American Holistic Medical Association. (Antioxidants

Potential Healing Power
May help: • **Protect against liver damage from alcohol, hepatitis and chemical toxins** • **Regenerate already damaged liver tissue**

counter the effects of naturally occurring toxins called free radicals.) "In animal studies, it has prevented liver damage, and in human studies, it has sped recovery from hepatitis," says Dr. Gaby.

Studies in Hungary, Germany and elsewhere demonstrate that silymarin holds promise for treating various liver disorders, including damage from exposure to chemical toxins and cirrhosis caused by alcohol abuse.

Don't Go It Alone

Who should reap the benefits of milk thistle, and how? First, don't fool around with liver problems. If you have hepatitis, cirrhosis or any other liver-related condition, see your doctor.

There have never been any reports of problems associated with milk thistle consumption, and some European physicians prescribe a standardized extract for liver disease. In the United States, this product, sometimes marketed under the name Thisilyn, is available as a food supplement.

A few American doctors also use milk thistle. Dr. Gaby, for example, recommends silymarin extract to some patients with chronic liver disease. He says he gets good results. "One man had elevated liver enzymes for six years—a sign of liver damage, in this case of unknown origin. Various liver specialists offered no help," he says. "But one month after he began taking silymarin regularly, the enzymes came down to normal levels and stayed there."

Traditionally, almost every part of the milk thistle has been used for food—even the leaves, with the spines removed. But the therapeutic substances in milk thistle are not water-soluble, so a tea would be ineffective, points out Varro E. Tyler, Ph.D., professor of pharmacognosy at Purdue University School of Pharmacy in West Lafayette, Indiana, and author of *The Honest Herbal*. And since silymarin is poorly absorbed by the human digestive system, he adds, capsules of concentrate are the only source of the compound that's effective.

If you want to take milk thistle products, it might be a good idea to discuss it with your doctor.

Mullein

The Velvety Respiratory Soother

Mullein (rhymes with sullen) is generally considered a minor medicinal herb. But James A. Duke, Ph.D., a botanist retired from the U.S. Depart-

Potential Healing Power

May help:
- Relieve coughs
- Reduce congestion
- Ease indigestion
- Soothe stings and scrapes

ment of Agriculture and author of *The CRC Handbook of Medicinal Herbs*, laments this status: "I'm a real believer in mullein," he explains. "Once my wife and I returned from a trip to China, and we both had bronchitis. She went to the doctor and did what he said. I took mullein tea. My bronchitis cleared up before hers did."

Mullein grows almost everywhere, and its velvety leaves, rodlike stem and striking yellow flowers are hard to miss. Mullein has a long history in herbal medicine. Its botanical family name—Scrophulariaceae—is derived from *scrofula*, an old term for chronically swollen lymph glands, later identified as a form of tuberculosis. Early on, this herb gained a reputation as a respiratory remedy. And physicians from India to England touted it as a remedy for coughs and chest congestion.

In a 1986 survey of folk medicine in Indiana, Varro E. Tyler, Ph.D., professor of pharmacognosy at Purdue University School of Pharmacy in West Lafayette, Indiana, and author of *The Honest Herbal*, discovered that the herb remains "very popular" for respiratory complaints.

Dr. Duke is not the only herb expert to value

mullein. Daniel B. Mowrey, Ph.D., director of the American Phytotherapy Research Laboratory in Salt Lake City, Utah, and author of *The Scientific Validation of Herbal Medicine*, says it soothes not only the respiratory tract but also the digestive system: "It's a shame there's been so little research on mullein. I think it's very valuable. For stings and scrapes while hiking, for example, crush a few leaves in your hand and apply it on the wound as a poultice. It's very soothing." However, like any hairy plant, mullein has the potential for being irritating. It is not likely that irritation will occur, but discontinue use if it does.

To brew a medicinal tea, use 1 to 2 teaspoons of dried leaves per cup of boiling water. Steep for ten minutes. Drink up to three cups per day. Mullein tastes bitter, so you might want to add sugar or honey and lemon, or mix it into an herbal beverage blend. In a tincture, take ½ to 1 teaspoon up to three times a day. There have been no reports of mullein causing adverse effects.

Oregano

It's Not Just for Pizza

Rumor has it that oregano didn't become a popular seasoning in the United States until after World War II, when soldiers who'd been stationed in the

Potential Healing Power

May help:
- Soothe coughs
- Aid digestion

Mediterranean returned home with a penchant for pizza.

Whether that's true or not, this pungent herb has been around for centuries, and many of its early uses were medicinal rather than culinary. The ancient Greeks made poultices from the leaves and used them to treat sores and aching muscles. Traditional Chinese doctors have used oregano for centuries to relieve fever, vomiting, diarrhea, jaundice and itchy skin. In Europe, the herb is still used to improve digestion and soothe coughs.

Little contemporary research has been done on the medical uses of oregano. The work that has been done shows that this herb contains two essential components, thymol and carvacol, which are also found in another herb, thyme.

Thymol can be used to help loosen phlegm in the lungs, according to Norman R. Farnsworth, Ph.D., director of the Program for Collaborative Research in the Pharmaceutical Sciences at the University of Illinois at Chicago.

In Germany, where herbal medicine is popular, syrups containing thymol are frequently prescribed for even the most serious kinds of coughs. In the United States, you're most likely to find thymol in cough remedies such as Vicks Menthol Cough Drops and in topical cough and cold products such as Vicks Va-poRub.

The ingredients in oregano that soothe coughs also help unknot muscles in the digestive tract. So there's some scientific basis for using this herb as a digestive aid, Dr. Farnsworth says. Oregano also has a reputation as a menstruation promoter. "Pregnant women may safely use this herb as a seasoning, but they should avoid taking large amounts," Dr. Farnsworth warns.

For a warm, spicy tea that can settle the stomach or soothe a cough, use one to two teaspoons of dried herb per cup of boiling water. Let it steep for ten minutes.

Peppermint

After-Dinner Digestive Aid

The fragrance and flavor of mint put a refreshing zing into thousands of products, from candy and chewing gum to cosmetics and medicines. But mint—in particular, peppermint—is more than just another pleasant taste. It lives up to its centuries-old reputation for easing indigestion and other ailments.

Today's custom of taking a mint after dinner is nothing new. The ancient Romans used mint after meals to aid digestion. Peppermint, a hybrid of other

Potential Healing Power

May help:
- Ease intestinal gas
- Relieve indigestion and diarrhea
- Reduce congestion
- Soothe muscle soreness
- Treat irritable bowel syndrome
- Calm menstrual cramps

mint species, is a relative newcomer, first identified in England around 1700. (Spearmint, a related plant, is also used for flavoring but is not considered medicinally potent like peppermint.) As early as 1801, American herbalists recommended peppermint preparations for gas, colic, hiccups and nausea.

"Peppermint is probably our best-known remedy for stomach problems," says Daniel B. Mowrey, Ph.D., director of the American Phytotherapy Research Laboratory in Salt Lake City, Utah, and author of *The Scientific Validation of Herbal Medicine*. The herb tames tummy trouble through several actions, he says: Its essential oils stimulate the gallbladder and encourage bile secretion while helping the muscles that line the stomach and intestines to function smoothly. Peppermint oil in extremely high concentrations may also inhibit and kill many microorganisms associated with digestive and other problems.

Peppermint can produce a relieving burp after a big, heavy meal or calm the crampiness of indigestion or diarrhea. In recent years, medical researchers have found peppermint helpful for irritable bowel syndrome, a common and hard-to-treat ailment with no known cause. The anti-spasmodic action of peppermint has also given the plant a possibly undeserved reputation for soothing menstrual cramps. Its effectiveness has not been proven.

The active ingredient that gives peppermint its kick is menthol—a potent aromatic chemical in the plant's volatile oil. Menthol (usually a synthetic version) is one of the pungent key ingredients in many popular products, from Vicks VapoRub to Noxzema. Mentholated remedies help clear congestion in the head and upper respiratory passages and, applied externally, help ease sore muscles and cool inflammation.

Tapping In to Menthol Power

Few herbal remedies are more innocuous than peppermint tea, which is widely available loose or in tea bags. It's a refreshing remedy enjoyed by thousands to relieve digestive upset. Peppermint candies are also a popular option, but these may not contain sufficient oil to actually be therapeutic. Peppermint oil is highly concentrated and should be used only in small, recommended amounts. (Pure menthol is poisonous, and should never be taken internally.)

Although peppermint is a time-honored remedy for colicky babies, some authorities discourage its use. "Don't give the tea to infants or very young children," counsels Varro E. Tyler, Ph.D., professor of pharmacognosy at Purdue University School of Pharmacy in West Lafayette, Indiana, and author of *The Honest Herbal*. "The menthol may give them a choking sensation." If you do give peppermint tea to older youngsters, make sure it's a very weak dilution.

Rosemary

Fragrant Cancer Fighter

In ancient Greece, students tucked sprigs of this spicy, pine-scented herb in their hair, supposedly to improve their ability to study. That's how rosemary came by its reputation as a memory sharpener.

That particular ability has yet to be proven, but other traditional uses for rosemary are holding up under scrutiny in the laboratory, and some additional benefits are being discovered as well.

Rosemary works so well at preventing fats from becoming rancid that the food industry sometimes uses extracts of rosemary oil as a food preservative. Rosemary oil is a strong antioxidant—which means it protects fats from being attacked by oxygen. Because oxygen damage is also known to be a factor in the development of cancer, researchers have been looking at its potential in this area as well.

Several studies done in the last several years show that oil from the leaves of the very plant sold as a spice for flavoring can help prevent the development of cancerous tumors in laboratory animals.

In one study, led by Chi-Tang Ho, Ph.D., professor in the Department of Food Science at Rutgers University in New Brunswick, New Jersey, applying rosemary oil to the skin of experimental animals reduced their risk of cancer to half that found in animals that did not receive the application of oil.

In other studies by the same research team, animals whose diets contained some rosemary oil had about half the incidence of colon cancer or lung cancer compared with animals not eating rosemary. And researchers at the University of Illinois in Urbana found that rosemary cut by half the incidence of breast cancer in animals at high risk for developing the disease.

"In the few studies done so far, rosemary has proven to be a strong inhibitor of the development and growth of cancerous tumors," says Dr. Ho. "Given orally or used topically, it has consistently reduced the incidence of cancer by about half." Further studies will demonstrate whether rosemary offers cancer protection to humans as well, he adds.

Like many culinary herbs, rosemary also helps to relax muscles, including the smooth muscles of the digestive tract and uterus. So it's sometimes used to soothe digestive upsets and relieve menstrual cramps. In large amounts, however, it appears to have the opposite effect—causing intestinal irritation and cramping. (In fact, larger doses of rosemary oil and other rosemary preparations can be a risk to pregnancy.)

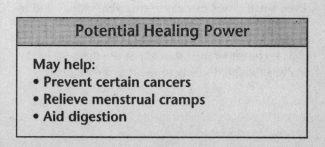

Potential Healing Power

May help:
- **Prevent certain cancers**
- **Relieve menstrual cramps**
- **Aid digestion**

Enjoying Rosemary

Rosemary makes a wonderful addition to meats such as pork, lamb, beef and chicken and can turn an ordinary pizza into a culinary masterpiece, especially when it's paired with a healthy dose of garlic. One holiday Italian bread combines rosemary and raisins in a braided eggbread that makes fragrant, delicious toast.

But is the small amount of rosemary you would typically use to season a dish enough to give you a therapeutic effect? Surprisingly, the answer may be yes.

"We've done studies that looked at both large amounts and smaller amounts in the diet and found benefits even with small amounts," Dr. Ho says. "When animals were fed a diet that contained 2 percent (by weight) of rosemary, we saw significant cancer protection. But when we cut that amount way back, to $\frac{1}{100}$ of that amount, rosemary still had a very strong effect. Even just using a fraction of a teaspoon a day could have potential health benefits."

If you prefer a tea, you can make a pleasant-tasting brew with one teaspoon of crushed dried leaves in a cup of boiling water. Let steep for ten minutes.

Avoid using rosemary oil in any amount, though. Even small doses can cause stomach, kidney and intestinal problems, and large amounts may be poisonous.

Pregnant women should not use the herb medicinally, although it's okay to use it as a seasoning.

Sage

A Potential Diabetes Fighter

You may recall the scene in *Zorba the Greek* where Anthony Quinn refuses an offer of sage tea and calls instead for rum. But other Greeks in Zorba's fictional world drank sage tea. And real-world Greeks do as well.

For centuries in Greece sage was believed to have medicinal value. As a tea it was thought to slow menstrual bleeding, while mixed with wine it was thought to stimulate menstruation. Throughout history sage has also been used as a muscle relaxant, an antiperspirant and a treatment for sore throats, diarrhea, venereal disease and a host of other conditions. It was also applied to wounds and insect bites.

The use of sage over time has been so extensive, in fact, that one text lists some 60-plus medical uses for it. Its Latin name—*Salvia officinalis*—seems appropriate, as it is derived from *salvere*, meaning "to heal or be healthy."

Sweet Relief

Does sage live up to its sterling reputation when medical science takes a look at it? In some ways, yes.

Because of its antiseptic qualities, sage does have merit as a gargle for sore throat, says Varro E. Tyler,

Potential Healing Power

May help:
- Soothe sore throat
- Fight diabetes

Ph.D., professor of pharmacognosy at Purdue University School of Pharmacy in West Lafayette, Indiana, and author of *The Honest Herbal*. In fact, it's used extensively for that purpose in Germany.

There's also compelling new research indicating that sage may be of value to people with diabetes. In Type II (non-insulin-dependent) diabetes, the hormone insulin does not work as efficiently as it should. Insulin has the job of helping the body's cells use glucose—the simple sugar your body uses as fuel. Laboratory studies indicate that sage may boost insulin's action, says Richard Anderson, Ph.D., lead scientist in vitamin and mineral nutrition at the U.S. Department of Agriculture's Human Nutrition Research Center in Beltsville, Maryland. Sage was among 24 herbs tested that were found to boost insulin activity two- to five-fold or more, says Dr. Anderson.

For people who have diabetes, this means that drinking sage tea in conjunction with their insulin treatments is worth a try, says Dr. Anderson. "It may be that they will need less insulin," he says.

The exact mechanism by which sage improves the activity of insulin is not yet known, and that's the next phase of research to be undertaken, says Dr. Anderson.

Putting Sage to Work

A person with diabetes can use sage any way that's convenient, says Dr. Anderson. You can use the herb as a spice or drink it as a tea, as long as you ingest it, he says.

To make a tea, pour a cup of boiling water over one to two teaspoons of dried leaves and steep for ten minutes. If you have diabetes, it would be a good idea to discuss using sage with your doctor.

For sore throat, allow the tea to cool till warm, then gargle as needed.

St.-John's-wort

A Natural Antidepressant

St.-John's-wort has been used in herbal healing for more than 2,000 years. Herbal healers thought they had a pretty good handle on what it can do, but its most exciting potential medical use was discovered in 1988. That's when researchers at New York University found that St.-John's-wort has dramatic action against the type of virus that causes acquired immune deficiency syndrome (AIDS). Since then, some AIDS patients have reported positive results using the herb, and a study sanctioned by the Food and Drug Admin-

Potential Healing Power
May help: • Fight AIDS • Heal burns • Relieve depression • Treat minor wounds

istration is under way, testing the effects of some of the herb's constituents in people who have AIDS.

Initial studies of St.-John's-wort have caused tremendous excitement among people with AIDS. Since early 1989, according to *AIDS Treatment News*, "almost all the reports we have heard from users have been good." And medical researchers are hopeful that within the next few years, a chemical component of St.-John's-wort (hypericin) will be used to treat AIDS.

"I'm very intrigued by hypericin," says Varro E. Tyler, Ph.D., professor of pharmacognosy at Purdue University School of Pharmacy in West Lafayette, Indiana, and author of *The Honest Herbal*. "Many AIDS drugs have not panned out, but everything I've heard about hypericin looks positive. I'm eager to see the results of the trial."

Wound Healer of Old

The leaves and flowers of St.-John's-wort contain special glands that release a red oil when pinched. Early Christians named the plant in honor of John the Baptist, because they believed it released its blood-red oil on August 29, the anniversary of the saint's beheading. (*Wort* is Old English for "plant.")

Perhaps because of its oil's blood-red color, St.-John's-wort has a long history of use as a wound treatment. Several scientific studies have confirmed this use. Medical researchers have found that St.-John's-wort does, in fact, contain antiviral, antibacterial and anti-inflammatory chemicals. One German study showed that, compared with conventional treatment, a St.-John's-wort ointment substantially cut the healing time of burns and caused less scarring. (This ointment is not available as an approved drug in the United States.)

That's not all the herb does, however. There's more.

"Initially, hypericin, one compound in St.-John's-wort, was considered the strong inhibitor of monoamine oxidase (MAO)," says Bernie Olin, Pharm.D., editor of *The Lawrence Review of Natural Products*, a St. Louis–based newsletter that summarizes scientific research on medicinal herbs. New studies suggest that two other constituents of St.-John's-wort, xanthones and flavonoids, are the active MAO inhibitors, which are an important class of anti-depressant medication. (Prescription MAO inhibitors include Nardil and Parnate.) In a small German study, six depressed women were given a St.-John's-wort preparation. "After six weeks," Dr. Olin explains, "they all showed improvement."

Tapping This Herb's Many Uses

To make an antidepressant tea, use one to two teaspoons of dried herb per cup of boiling water. Steep 10 to 15 minutes. Drink up to three cups a day. St.-John's-wort tastes initially sweet, then bitter and astringent.

After eating large quantities of St.-John's-wort, cattle often develop severe sunburn with blistering (photosensitization). Several sources say the same is true for humans, especially those with fair skin. If you have fair skin, use St.-John's-wort cautiously, and wear protective clothing when you're out in the sun.

For AIDS, St.-John's-wort should only be taken under the guidance of a physician. The preparation used is not the bulk herb but rather a standardized hypericin extract. People with AIDS say the herb is relatively nontoxic, but some have reported sun sensitivity, drowsiness, nausea and diarrhea.

For wound treatment, apply crushed leaves and flowers to the affected area.

Saw Palmetto

Promise for Prostate Problems

Young men don't want to think about it. Older men don't want to talk about it. But the reality is that more than half of all men over age 50 will experience the discomfort of an enlarged prostate gland.

In the not-too-distant past men sometimes relied on remedies made from saw palmetto berries for relief.

These days there are more treatment options available—usually prescription drugs or surgery—but a man can *still* seek relief from saw palmetto. The only difference these days is that the herb increasingly has the blessing of modern medical science.

What exactly is this prostate unpleasantness that so many men have to deal with? The prostate is a tiny gland located at the base of a man's bladder. It completely encircles the urethra—the narrow tube through which urine exits the body. When the gland enlarges as a man ages, it sometimes blocks the urethra, creating a frequent, urgent need to urinate, a weak or interrupted flow and difficulty emptying the bladder.

Berries versus Blockage

Saw palmetto is a palm that grows throughout the southeastern United States, and its therapeutic value lies in its dark red berries.

The herb's active ingredient is unknown. But studies done in Europe show that an extract from the berries appears to counteract the effects of androgens, male sex hormones that may cause prostate enlargement, says Varro E. Tyler, Ph.D., professor of pharmacognosy at Purdue University School of Pharmacy in West Lafayette, Indiana, and author of *The Honest*

Potential Healing Power

May help:
• Improve symptoms of enlarged prostate

Herbal. In Europe, Dr. Tyler notes, medications based on saw palmetto are routinely prescribed for enlarged prostate.

Saw palmetto products are available in this country, although they are not labeled for use in treating an enlarged prostate. That's because the Food and Drug Administration (FDA) has banned marketing saw palmetto medications for this problem, claiming there is too little proof that they work. The FDA evidently "overlooked" the European research when it made that ruling, notes Dr. Tyler.

But the FDA did not ban saw palmetto here; it simply restricted marketing claims. In fact, some American health practitioners and herbalists recommend the herb highly.

"I recommend saw palmetto berry extract for men with enlarged prostate glands," says Alan R. Gaby, M.D., a Baltimore physician who practices nutritional and natural medicine and is president of the American Holistic Medical Association. "Studies have shown that it can improve urinary flow rates and reduce symptoms like urinary hesitancy and weak flow. In many cases, it works as well or better than the prescription drug—and it's cheaper and safer."

No Substitute for the Doctor

Just because some herbalists believe saw palmetto works doesn't mean you should use it on your own. Dr. Gaby and other herb experts caution against self-medicating for an enlarged prostate.

Seeking medical care for prostate symptoms can be a lifesaver, points out Dr. Gaby. "Taking this or any herb does not eliminate the need for older men to get a routine checkup for prostate cancer," he says. Alert your doctor if you take any saw palmetto product, he warns, because the herb may change the results of blood tests that are used to detect prostate cancer. It's also inadvisable to take saw palmetto products plus prescription medication for an enlarged prostate, he adds. They could interact.

Finally, the form in which you take the herb is important, says Dr. Tyler. An oil-based extract was used in the scientific studies. "A water-based saw palmetto preparation, such as a tea, would give little or no benefit," says Dr. Tyler.

If you want to take saw palmetto, use an extract prepared by a reputable herbal medicine company and follow dosage directions on the package. The commonly recommended dose is 320 milligrams of oil-based extract daily. And make sure you discuss it with your doctor.

Senna

A Powerful Laxative

During the ninth century, legend has it, the great caliph of Baghdad became dissatisfied with the medicines available in his court, particularly the laxatives. It seems they did more harm than good, causing severe abdominal distress. The caliph sent for a famous physician, Mesue the Elder, who brought

Potential Healing Power

May help:
• Relieve constipation

new medicines to the court, including a "gentler" laxative, senna.

If senna was the gentler alternative, the caliph's old laxatives must have been real gut-wrenchers. Senna is such a powerful laxative that it can cause cramping and abdominal distress if not used with caution.

"Like aloe, buckthorn and cascara sagrada, senna contains anthraquinone glycosides, chemicals that stimulate the colon," says James A. Duke, Ph.D., a botanist retired from the U.S. Department of Agriculture and author of *The CRC Handbook of Medicinal Herbs*.

It's quite possible that you've taken small doses of senna without being aware of it. The herb is an ingredient in many over-the-counter laxatives, including Fletcher's Castoria, Senokot, Perdiem and Innerclean Herbal Laxative.

Anthraquinone laxatives should be considered as treatment for constipation only as a last resort, says Anne Simons, M.D., assistant clinical professor of family and community medicine at the University of California's San Francisco Medical Center. "First, eat a diet that's higher in fiber, drink more fluids and get more exercise," she recommends. "If that doesn't provide relief, try a bulk-forming laxative." One such laxative is psyllium (Metamucil). "If that doesn't help," advises Dr. Simons, "try ingesting the lubricant laxative mineral oil. And if that doesn't provide relief, try an anthraquinone laxative in consultation with your physician."

Senna is certainly effective, but most authorities consider two other anthraquinone laxatives to be gentler—buckthorn and cascara sagrada.

A Moving Experience

Senna tastes awful. Herbalists generally discourage using the plant material and instead recommend over-the-counter products containing it. However, if you're interested in trying the unprocessed herb, you can brew a medicinal tea from one to two teaspoons of dried leaves per cup of boiling water. Let steep for ten minutes. Add sugar, honey and lemon to taste. You can also mix it with pleasant-tasting herbs, such as anise, fennel, peppermint, chamomile, ginger, coriander or licorice. Drink up to one cup a day in the morning or before bed for no more than a few days. To take senna in capsule form, simply follow the package directions.

Senna should not be given to children under two. For older children and people over 65, start with a low-strength preparation and increase strength if necessary.

Don't, under any circumstances, be tempted to use more than these small amounts of senna. Larger doses can cause diarrhea, nausea and severe abdominal cramping, with possible dehydration. Senna's powerful action means it should not be used by those with chronic gastrointestinal conditions, such as ulcers, colitis or hemorrhoids. Pregnant and nursing women should not take senna. And senna should never be used for more than two weeks, because over time, it can cause what's known as lazy bowel syndrome—the inability to move stool without chemical stimulation.

Slippery Elm

Early American Throat Soother

When alumni come to visit the University of Connecticut School of Pharmacy in Storrs, John Michael Edwards, Ph.D., is more than happy to show them around the old alma mater. But all the while he's got at least one eye on the department's jar of slippery elm.

It seems that the graduates developed a taste for the stuff when they were students—and they aren't afraid to raid the jar when they're back in town, says Dr. Edwards, associate dean of the school of pharmacy.

"In the old days, the pharmacy students had to be able not only to identify powdered drugs but to identify them in chunks—and slippery elm was one of them," says Dr. Edwards. "And if you suck on a piece of slippery elm, you get this mucilage out of it that's sort of sweet. Every so often, we have an alumnus who comes back and pounces on the jar of slippery elm bark."

Former pharmacy students aren't the first to covet slippery elm bark. Before Dutch elm disease decimated the great slippery elm forests of the northeastern United States, this plant was perhaps the country's favorite home remedy—used in sore throat lozenges and as a hot cereal like oatmeal for ulcers, heartburn and common digestive complaints.

That sweet mucilage apparently coats and soothes mucous membranes. "There's a polysaccharide in the bark that's very soothing, there's no question about that," says Christopher W. W. Beecher, Ph.D., associate professor of pharmacognosy in the Department of Medicinal Chemistry and Pharmacognosy at the University of Illinois at Chicago. A polysaccharide is a kind of carbohydrate.

Soothing Relief

You don't have to scout the forests for slippery elm trees to take advantage of this old-fashioned herb. You

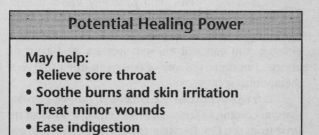

Potential Healing Power

May help:
• Relieve sore throat
• Soothe burns and skin irritation
• Treat minor wounds
• Ease indigestion

can still buy slippery elm throat lozenges in health food stores and some drugstores.

If you prefer a pleasant-tasting tea, add a cup of boiling water to a teaspoon of slippery elm powder or to slippery elm tea that you can buy at a health food store. Add sugar or honey to taste.

For a poultice to pack on burns, boils, minor wounds and inflamed skin, simply add enough water to slippery elm powder to create a paste. Some people are allergic to slippery elm. If you find that the paste irritates your skin, discontinue use.

Tarragon

Anti-cancer Activist

Although tarragon has a long and venerable history as a healing plant, you probably know it as a kitchen herb—the pretty, green, spiky-looking plant that's used in expensive bottles of tarragon vinegar. You can still enjoy it just for its flavor, of course, but there's plenty of reason to think of it as a therapeutic agent as well.

Tarragon contains 72 potential cancer preventives, according to James A. Duke, Ph.D., a botanist retired from the U.S. Department of Agriculture and author of *The CRC Handbook of Medicinal Herbs*. The herb's main cancer-blocking punch comes from a chemical called caffeic acid, which has the ability to cleanse the body of naturally occurring harmful substances known as free radicals. Caffeic acid also has some ability to kill viruses. "Caffeic acid is one ingredient in tarragon I would seek if I were looking to prevent cancer, flu or herpes," says Dr. Duke.

Help for Herpes

"If I had herpes I would be drinking lemon balm tea with tarragon in it, and I would be applying the tea bag to the blisters," says Dr. Duke. "Both have antiviral activity, and I'm a great believer in synergy." Besides, tarragon will add a pleasant flavor to the tea, he says.

For relief from either oral or genital herpes, you can try a cup of tea with a lemon balm tea bag and one teaspoon of dried tarragon. (You can purchase lemon balm tea in many health food stores.) Let the brew steep for 10 to 15 minutes before drinking. Drink up to three cups a day.

Potential Healing Power

May help:
• Prevent certain cancers
• Heal herpes outbreaks
• Fight flu

Tea

A Cup of Comfort

I t's the world's most popular herbal remedy and the second most popular beverage, after water. Technically, any concoction of plants steeped in water is a tea. But when most people say "tea," they mean the bracing brew beloved by everyone from Chinese peasants to the English aristocracy: the fragrant leaves of an Asian evergreen shrub called *Camellia sinensis*. Several related species are also known simply as tea.

As it happens, a nice cup of tea may give you more than just a morning lift. Research suggests that tea, especially the green tea popular in the Orient, may have beneficial actions against heart disease and cancer.

Caffeine Plus

Tea contains several stimulant compounds, including caffeine and theophylline. An average cup of tea contains between 10 and 50 milligrams of caffeine, depending on the type of tea and the preparation method. (By comparison, a cup of brewed coffee has about 100 milligrams.) Both caffeine and theophylline act as bronchodilators, agents that can help open clogged respiratory passages. So your grandmother was right if she gave you hot tea to ease the misery of colds, flu or bronchitis.

There's no firm evidence that caffeine in moderation poses any risk to most people, although in excess, it can cause jitters and insomnia.

The Green Scene

Recently, scientists have been finding that tea may offer broader health benefits. Mostly, their research has been on green tea, a type more popular in the Orient than in the United States, where black tea is the leading seller. Green tea supplies generous amounts of substances called polyphenols, including one called catechin. Black tea leaves, which undergo an added process of fermentation, contain less catechin.

There's a small but growing body of evidence that the catechin and some related substances in green tea may have cancer-fighting properties.

For example, one research team found that catechin derived from a traditional Himalayan tea helped prevent skin tumors in laboratory animals. Other studies using laboratory animals have shown that green tea has a protective effect against tumors of the lung, stomach and liver. Can humans reap the same benefits? Only more research will tell, say the experts.

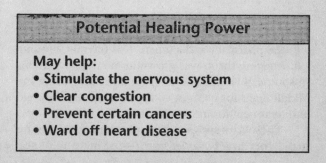

Potential Healing Power

May help:
- Stimulate the nervous system
- Clear congestion
- Prevent certain cancers
- Ward off heart disease

Tea for the Heart

It's well established that moderate tea drinking does no harm to the heart, and it may do some good.

An Israeli study of more than 5,000 tea drinkers found a link between tea consumption and lower blood cholesterol, although the cause-and-effect relationship wasn't clear. Japanese researchers, however, found that green tea polyphenols seemed to lower blood cholesterol and blood pressure in laboratory animals.

Researchers have also found that tea is a mild diuretic, helping to rid the body of excess fluid.

To enjoy the multiple benefits of tea—including its wonderful taste—simply buy a commercial product and follow the directions on the package.

Thyme

Ace Antiseptic

Thyme has a centuries-long history of use, in both the pharmacy and kitchen. This fragrant, ground-hugging shrub was grown in monastery gardens in southern France and in Spain and Italy during the Middle Ages for use as a cough remedy, digestive aid and treatment for intestinal parasites.

These days sprigs of its pungent, minty leaves are mandatory in a *bouquet garni*—the mixture of seasonings used to spice up just about every French food from soup to salad.

And the herb is still being used for medicinal purposes. A solution of thyme's most active ingredient, thymol, is used in many over-the-counter products, including Listerine mouthwash and Vicks VapoRub. "Thymol is added to these products because of its well-known antibacterial and antifungal properties," explains Brian M. Lawrence, Ph.D., a research scientist and editor of the *Journal of Essential Oil Research*.

Thymol apparently also has a therapeutic effect on the lungs. "The oil from the leaves of this plant, when ingested or inhaled, helps to loosen phlegm and relax the muscles in the respiratory tract," explains Norman R. Farnsworth, Ph.D., director of the Program for Collaborative Research in the Pharmaceutical Sciences at the University of Illinois at Chicago.

In Germany, where herbal medicine is considerably more mainstream than it is in the United States, concoctions of thyme are frequently prescribed for coughs, including those resulting from whooping cough, bronchitis and emphysema. In the United States, thyme extract was included in a popular cough syrup, Pertussin, that is no longer on the market. "These days, you are most

Potential Healing Power

May help:
• Kill bacteria and fungi
• Loosen phlegm
• Relieve coughs

likely to find thyme in 'cold formula' herbal teas or remedies for coughs that are distributed by small companies and sold at health food stores," Dr. Farnsworth says.

Taking Thyme

To use thyme safely and effectively, brew a tea or infusion, Dr. Farnsworth suggests. Use two teaspoons of dried herb per cup of boiling water and steep for ten minutes.

The Food and Drug Administration includes thyme on its list of herbs generally regarded as safe. "As with many herbs, though, too large a dose may produce intestinal problems," Dr. Farnsworth warns. If you experience diarrhea or bloating, cut back on the amount you're using or discontinue use altogether. And make sure you take thyme as tea, not as oil. Undiluted thyme oil can be toxic, causing headache, nausea, vomiting and weakness, as well as thyroid, heart and lung problems.

Turmeric

India's Amazing Medicinal Plant

Most Americans are only vaguely aware of turmeric as an ingredient in Indian curry. We certainly don't think of it as a healing herb. Indians do, however.

A great deal of scientific research—almost all of it Indian—shows that turmeric aids digestion, prevents ulcers, protects the liver, helps prevent heart disease and may one day be used to treat cancer.

A relative of ginger, turmeric has held a place of honor in India's traditional Ayurvedic medicine for thousands of years. It was used as a digestive aid and treatment for fever, wounds, infections, dysentery, arthritis, jaundice and other liver problems. The Chinese adopted turmeric and used it similarly.

"Turmeric stimulates the flow of bile," says Pi-Kwang Tsung, Ph.D., former assistant professor of pathology at the University of Connecticut Medical School in Farmington and currently editor of *The East-West Medical Digest*. "This means it helps digest fats, confirming its traditional use as a digestive herb."

"Turmeric has strong liver-protective properties," agrees Bernie Olin, Pharm.D., editor of *The Lawrence Review of Natural Products*, a St. Louis–based newsletter that summarizes scientific research on med-

Potential Healing Power

May help:
- Aid digestion
- Relieve arthritis
- Treat dysentery
- Protect the liver
- Combat heart disease
- Ward off ulcers
- Prevent certain cancers

icinal herbs. If you drink alcohol regularly and/or take high doses of many pharmaceutical drugs—including the common pain reliever acetaminophen (Tylenol)—medical researchers say you may be at risk for liver damage. Using turmeric may offer a degree of protection.

The latest studies show that turmeric also protects the stomach lining and helps prevent ulcers, says Alan R. Gaby, M.D., a Baltimore physician who practices nutritional and natural medicine and is president of the American Holistic Medical Association. "Turmeric's anti-ulcer effect should be cause for celebration among curry lovers with Type-A personalities, like myself." And several studies show that curcumin, an active chemical in turmeric, has anti-inflammatory action, lending credence to the herb's traditional use in treating arthritis.

Like most culinary herbs, turmeric helps retard food spoilage because it has antibacterial action. In laboratory tests, turmeric also fights protozoa—microbes that cause a multitude of human ills. These tests lend credence to the herb's traditional use in treating dysentery, which is caused by this type of microorganism.

Powerful Protection

Several medical studies now suggest that turmeric may also help prevent heart disease by lowering cholesterol and preventing the formation of the internal blood clots that trigger heart attack (and many strokes). These findings come from studies done with laboratory animals and cannot necessarily be applied to people. But turmeric is a tasty spice that does no harm, and these studies suggest it might do some real good.

After a while, you begin to wonder if there's anything turmeric *can't* do. Sure enough, it even has potential as a cancer fighter. Several studies on laboratory animals show that curcumin has anti-cancer activity, probably because it is a powerful antioxidant. (Antioxidants are substances that counteract naturally occurring toxic substances called free radicals.)

Evidence from a recent study, a human trial in smokers, makes this herb look even more beneficial. Smokers' urine contains substances (mutagens) that cause genetic mutation. Mutagens are often carcinogens, or cancer causers. Indian researchers added 1.5 grams of turmeric a day (about a teaspoon) to the diet of 16 smokers for a month. The result was a significant reduction in urinary mutagens.

Giving Turmeric a Try

Since Indian research shows that even a teaspoon of turmeric has medicinal value, it makes a lot of sense to enjoy turmeric as the Indians do—as a seasoning in foods. Turmeric tastes pleasant, but in large amounts it becomes somewhat bitter.

If you'd prefer to make a medicinal drink to aid digestion and possibly help prevent heart disease, use one teaspoon of turmeric powder per cup of warm milk. Drink up to three cups a day. Unusually large amounts of turmeric may cause stomach upset. If you find the drink doesn't agree with you, discontinue its use.

Ulcers, arthritis, liver disease, heart disease and cancer all require professional treatment. If you'd like to use turmeric in addition to standard therapies, discuss it with your doctor.

Medicinal turmeric preparations should not be given to children under two. For older children and people over 65, start with low-strength preparations and increase strength if necessary.

Valerian

A Safe Aid to Slumber

Valerian smells funky—sort of like a forgotten washrag left in a basement corner. And it tastes funny . . . as you might imagine sucking on that washrag *would* taste. (Cats don't share this view. They think valerian is the hottest thing since catnip.) Taste notwithstanding, herbalists for hundreds of years have relied on the woody roots of valerian to calm the anxious and relax the sleepless. But does it really work?

Numerous studies have shown that valerian does indeed help people with insomnia get to sleep faster and sleep better—without the groggy "morning-after" effects of standard prescription sedatives. No one is quite certain how valerian performs this magic.

"According to the latest information available, we simply don't know what the active ingredients are," says Varro E. Tyler, Ph.D., professor of pharmacognosy at Purdue University School of Pharmacy in West Lafayette, Indiana, and author of *The Honest Herbal*.

Chemicals in valerian called valepotriates act as muscle relaxants, making the herb potentially useful against menstrual cramps and other types of spasms. But even valerian preparations *without* valepotriates help slumbertime come faster—raising the possibility that some still-unidentified chemical, or a synergistic reaction among various compounds in the root, may confer its calming action.

Smart Use

In Europe, where herbal preparations are part of mainstream medicine, there are dozens of valerian preparations available to treat nervousness and insomnia. In this country, the root is available in the form of teas, tinctures, capsules and extracts.

Since the herb has a good record of safety, with few reported side effects, many herbalists—and a few doctors—suggest trying it if you toss and turn at night.

"I recommend it to my patients, and they say it helps," says Alan R. Gaby, M.D., a Baltimore physician who practices nutritional and natural medicine and is president of the American Holistic Medical Associa-

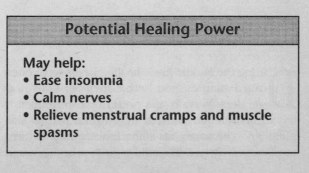

Potential Healing Power

May help:
• Ease insomnia
• Calm nerves
• Relieve menstrual cramps and muscle spasms

tion. "For some people, only the big guns—the prescription tranquilizers—will offer relief," he adds. "But for those with mild insomnia, it's the first thing I try, usually in capsule form." Simply follow the directions on the package. When using a tincture or extract, one teaspoon daily is the usual recommended dose. If taken as a tea, one cup should be sufficient.

As with any herbal remedy, be cautious about using large amounts over a long period, especially if you're using concentrated extracts; valerian in high doses has been reported to cause headaches and grogginess.

An important note: Don't be confused by the similarity of the herb's name to Valium. Valium is one of those "big gun" prescription sedatives. This powerful drug has no relation to valerian and should be used only under the strict supervision of a physician.

Vervain

A Neglected Tonic

During the Middle Ages, healing herbs were often called simples, and herbalists were known as simplers. Vervain was prescribed so frequently for so many conditions, it became known as simpler's joy. The name has some basis in fact. It turns out that vervain acts like mild aspirin, relieving minor pains and inflammation. It also has mild antidepressant effects.

In Egyptian mythology, vervain grew from the tears of Isis, goddess of fertility, as she grieved for her murdered brother/husband, Osiris. A thousand years later, vervain entered Christian mythology as the herb pressed into Christ's wounds to stanch his bleeding, hence one of its names, herb-of-the-cross.

Vervain has been used medicinally for thousands of years. Hippocrates recommended it for fever and plague. The twelfth-century German abbess and herbalist Hildegard of Bingen prescribed a medicinal tea of vervain and vermouth for "toxic blood" (infections), toothache and "discharges from the brain to the teeth." Our word *vervain* comes from the Celtic *ferfaen*, from *fer-*, "to drive away," and *-faen*, "stone"—a reference to its traditional use in treating kidney stones.

The Rodney Dangerfield of Herbs

In modern times, vervain has fallen by the medicinal wayside because its actions are mild. "But that's no reason to neglect this herb," says Daniel B. Mowrey, Ph.D., director of the American Phytotherapy Research Laboratory in Salt Lake City, Utah, and author of *The*

Potential Healing Power
May help: • Aid digestion • Relieve depression • Thwart headache • Ease minor aches and pains

Scientific Validation of Herbal Medicine. "It's a valuable tonic. Unfortunately, tonics don't get much respect in American pharmacology."

A tonic is a substance that doesn't have a dramatic action, but over time, its subtle effects strengthen the body and contribute to vitality. Vervain, Dr. Mowrey says, is slightly astringent, which helps digestion. It's mildly pain-relieving and anti-inflammatory, so it helps control minor aches and pains. Vervain has mild laxative action to help keep the digestive tract running smoothly. And it's a mild antidepressant, so it may improve mood, says Dr. Mowrey. No wonder medieval herbalists called vervain simpler's joy.

To make an infusion to treat headache, mild arthritis and other minor pains, use 2 teaspoons of dried herb per cup of boiling water. Steep for 10 to 15 minutes. Drink up to three cups a day. You can mask vervain's bitter taste with sugar, honey and lemon, or mix it with some other herbal beverage tea. If you buy a tincture, use ½ to 1 teaspoon up to three times a day.

White Willow

Herbal Aspirin

Mention "willow," and most people say "weeping." But the graceful tree should actually be seen as a source of joy. White willow is Nature's aspirin. In fact, pharmaceutical aspirin was originally created from a chemical very similar to one found in white willow bark.

Today there are more reasons than ever to use this herb. Medical research shows that this chemical in white willow (called salicin) not only reduces fever and relieves pain and inflammation but also may help prevent heart attack, stroke, digestive tract cancers and migraine headaches.

Chinese physicians have used willow to relieve pain since ancient times, but it took 2,000 years for this use to catch on in the West—an event that occurred almost by accident.

During the mid-1700s, British minister/physician Edmund Stone was trying to find a cheap substitute for cinchona bark, the rare, costly South American herb used to treat malaria (and later shown to contain the antimalarial drug, quinine). Cinchona was a bitter-tasting bark, and near Stone's Oxfordshire home, he found another bark that looked and tasted similar—white willow. As an experiment, he gave willow bark tea to people with fevers. Their fevers and pain subsided.

Potential Healing Power

May help:
- Reduce fever
- Relieve pain and inflammation
- Ward off heart attack and stroke
- Combat certain cancers
- Prevent migraine headache

Never mind that by today's scientific standards, Stone's experiment left a great deal to be desired. The thermometers of his day were so crude that he couldn't be sure if his subjects really had fevers to begin with. Nonetheless, the herb quickly became the treatment of choice for fever and subsequently for pain and inflammation as well.

During the early nineteenth century, European chemists created aspirin from white willow bark's active chemical—salicin. Aspirin hit the market for the first time in 1899, and within a few years, it was one of the most popular drugs on earth.

Bark Still Packs a Punch

Herbal experts say that white willow bark will work on almost anything you take aspirin for—most likely, fever, pain and inflammation. It will stand in for aspirin, but perhaps not quite as well.

"The salicylate content of willow bark varies considerably," says Varro E. Tyler, Ph.D., professor of pharmacognosy at Purdue University School of Pharmacy in West Lafayette, Indiana, and author of *The Honest Herbal*. "You may need several cups of white willow bark tea to approach the effectiveness of two standard aspirin tablets."

Recent studies show that taking about half an aspirin a day can significantly reduce risk of heart attack and stroke by reducing the likelihood of the internal blood clots that trigger these medical emergencies. Studies of aspirin's effectiveness have not been duplicated for willow bark, but Dr. Tyler says that in the body, "they become the same thing, salicylic acid."

The problem with using willow bark to prevent heart attack and stroke is uncertainty about the herb's salicin content. "But the preventive dose is quite low," Dr. Tyler says. "Many willow bark samples should contain enough. If you have a willow bark sample that helps reduce pain, it probably contains enough salicin to produce aspirin's preventive benefits."

James A. Duke, Ph.D., a botanist retired from the U.S. Department of Agriculture and author of *The CRC Handbook of Medicinal Herbs*, agrees: "I have used willow bark for toothache pain, and if I were at risk, I would drink willow bark tea for heart attack prevention." How much is enough? Given adequate salicin content, a cup or two a day should be enough, says Dr. Duke.

According to American Cancer Society researchers, the same low aspirin dose that helps prevent heart attack and stroke also significantly reduces deaths from four digestive tract cancers: tumors of the esophagus, stomach, colon and rectum. According to Dr. Tyler, if willow bark contains enough salicin, it should produce the same effects.

The herb may also help people who suffer from migraine headaches, since use of low-dose aspirin has been shown to significantly reduce attacks.

Brewing Up Some Bark

To take advantage of the healing powers of white willow bark, soak one teaspoon of powdered bark per cup of cold water for eight hours. Strain it and drink up to three cups a day. White willow tastes bitter and astringent. To improve the taste, you can add sugar or honey and lemon. You can also mix it into an herbal beverage tea.

Aspirin upsets some people's stomachs, but most herbalists say white willow bark rarely causes this problem. If stomach upset, nausea or ringing in the ears develops, reduce your dose or discontinue use. Pregnant women and those with chronic gastrointestinal conditions such as ulcers, colitis or Crohn's disease should not use this herb.

When children under 18 who have colds, flu or chicken pox take aspirin, they are at risk for Reye's syndrome, a potentially fatal condition. White willow has never been linked to Reye's syndrome, but because of its aspirin-like action, do not give it to children with fevers from those conditions. For complaints not involving fever, start children over 2 on low-strength preparations and increase strength if necessary. People over 65 should also begin with low-strength preparations.

Heart attack, stroke, cancer and migraines are serious conditions requiring professional care. If you'd like to use white willow bark in addition to standard therapies, discuss it with your doctor.

Wild Cherry

An Airway Cleaner

Early colonial settlers didn't have the option of running down to the corner drugstore for cough syrup or an expectorant when their kids had a cold. Instead, they stripped bark from a wild cherry tree, steeped it in hot water and offered it to their children as a hot, soothing beverage.

Today, not much has changed. Parents can run down to the corner drugstore for a bottle of cough syrup, all right. But chances are that the bottle is still going to contain wild cherry.

"Wild cherry is a flavoring agent that has a slight expectorant activity," says James E. Robbers, Ph.D., professor of pharmacognosy in the Department of Medicinal Chemistry and Pharmacognosy at Purdue University in West Lafayette, Indiana, and editor of the *Journal of Natural Products*. It contains benzaldehyde, a substance that loosens phlegm.

Generally, other ingredients with a more intense chemical activity are included in wild cherry cough syrups to boost the cherry's natural abilities and to provide the actual cough suppressant, says Dr. Robbers.

Loosening Things Up

Although the bottled variety of wild cherry cough syrup is more effective than wild cherry tea, the tea can be soothing to someone who's not feeling well.

If you'd like to make some tea, place one teaspoonful of wild cherry bark or leaves in a cup of boiling water. Steep for ten minutes and strain. Add honey, sugar or lemon to taste and enjoy. When using a tincture, follow the package directions.

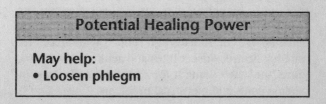

Potential Healing Power

May help:
• Loosen phlegm

Just two caveats: Do not give wild cherry tea to children under age two, and do not drink more than three cups a day. Wild cherry leaves, bark and fruit pits all contain hydrocyanic acid, which can be toxic in large amounts.

Witch Hazel

The Herb Even Doctors Recommend

Witch hazel is a popular home remedy for cuts, bruises, hemorrhoids and sore muscles. More than a million gallons of witch hazel water are sold each year in the United States, making it one of the nation's most widely used healing herbs. But ironically, commercial witch hazel water would be just as effective without its witch hazel.

Despite this herb's name, witch hazel has nothing to do with witchcraft. In medieval English, *witch* was spelled *wych*, and it meant flexible. Witch hazel is a tree with branches that are indeed flexible—so springy, in fact, that American Indians used them to make bows. The Indians also rubbed witch hazel tea on cuts, bruises, insect bites and aching muscles and joints, and they drank it for a variety of ailments, including colds and menstrual problems.

During the 1840s, an Indian medicine man introduced the herb's astringent properties to Theron T. Pond of Utica, New York, who began marketing it. Witch hazel water has been with us ever since.

The Astringent That Isn't

Early witch hazel water was simply tea on a large scale. This herb is high in astringent tannins, which dissolved in water-based witch hazel preparations, thus making them effective astringents. But about a century ago, manufacturers switched to steam distillation, a simpler process but one that eliminated the tannins—and all herbal astringent benefits. Nonetheless, Americans kept on using witch hazel water and swearing by it as a treatment for cuts, rashes and hemorrhoids.

Today it can be found in any pharmacy. "It's the active ingredient in Tucks hemorrhoid pads," says James A. Duke, Ph.D., a botanist retired from the U.S. Department of Agriculture and author of *The CRC Handbook of Medicinal Herbs*.

How can tannin-free witch hazel water have astringent benefits? "Witch hazel water isn't water anymore. It's 14 percent alcohol, which is also astringent," says Varro E. Tyler, Ph.D., professor of pharmacognosy

Potential Healing Power
May help: • Soothe skin irritation • Heal minor wounds • Treat hemorrhoids

at Purdue University School of Pharmacy in West Lafayette, Indiana, and author of *The Honest Herbal*.

If you want to get the astringent benefits of natural witch hazel, you'll have to brew up a batch yourself. Boil one teaspoon of powdered leaves or twigs per cup of water for ten minutes. Strain and cool. Apply the solution directly or mix it into an ointment.

The medical literature contains no reports of harm from external use of witch hazel. But if witch hazel causes minor discomforts, such as skin irritation, dilute it or discontinue use.